Grammatical Disorders in Aphasia

A Neurolinguistic Perspective

D1444366

Grammatical Disorders in Aphasia

A Neurolinguistic Perspective

edited by

ROELIEN BASTIAANSE

University of Groningen

and

YOSEF GRODZINSKY

Tel Aviv University

W

WHURR PUBLISHERS

LONDON AND PHILADELPHIA

First published 2000 by Whurr Publishers Ltd
19b Compton Terrrace
London N1 2UN
England
© 2000 Whurr Publishers Ltd

Reprinted 2002 and 2003

British Library Cataloguing in Publication Data
A catalogue record for this book is available from the
British Library.

ISBN 1 86156 135 0

Printed and bound in the UK by Publish on Demand
Limited, Highbury, London

Contents

Acknowledgements

All chapters in this book have been written by participants of the workshop *Grammatical Disorders in Aphasia*, held in Groningen, The Netherlands in the early summer of 1997, where work in progress was discussed by the researchers. This workshop was sponsored financially by several Dutch institutions; without this support, it would not have been possible to hold this meeting. We therefore gratefully acknowledge the grants of the Center for Language and Cognition Groningen (CLCG), Groningen Graduate School for Behavioural and Cognitive Neurosciences (BCN), Koninklijke Nederlandse Academie voor Wetenschappen (KNAW: Royal Dutch Academy of Sciences), Nederlandse Hartstichting (NHS: Dutch Heart Foundation), Nederlandse Organisatie voor Wetenschappelijk Onderzoek (NWO: Dutch Organization for Scientific Research), Stichting Afasie Nederland (SAN: Dutch Aphasia Foundation) and Stichting Groninger Universiteitsfonds (GUF: Groningen University Foundation). Yosef Grodzinsky was supported by NIDCD grant CD-00081 to the Aphasia Research Center, Department of Neurology, Boston University School of Medicine, and by the Israel-U.S. Binational Science Foundation grant 97-00451 to Tel Aviv University.

We would also like to thank the ASHA, who granted permission to republish the introductory chapter from Shapiro, An Introduction to Syntax; this paper was originally in the *Journal of Speech, Language and Hearing Research* 40: 254–72, in April 1997.

Roelien Bastiaanse
Yosef Grodzinsky

Contributors

Dr Jennifer Balogh
Aphasia Research Center
Boston VA Medical Center
USA
and
Department of Psychology
University of California, San Diego
USA

Prof Dr Roelien Bastiaanse
Department of Linguistics
University of Groningen
The Netherlands
and
Rehabilitation Center Het
Roessingh
Enschede, The Netherlands

Dr Vicky Bouck
Department of Psychology
University of California, San Diego
USA

Dr Susan Edwards
Department of Linguistic Science
University of Reading
United Kingdom

Dr Na'ama Friedmann
Department of Psychology
Tel Aviv University
Israel

Prof Dr Yosef Grodzinsky
Department of Psychology
Tel Aviv University
Israel
and
Aphasia Research Center
Boston VA Medical Center
USA

Dr Lea Ann Hald
Department of Psychology
University of Arizona, Tucson
USA

Dr Roal Jonkers
Faculty of Letters
University of Groningen
The Netherlands

Katalin Kiss, MA
Research Institute for Linguistics
Hungarian Academy of Sciences
Budapest
Hungary

Dr Tracy Love
Department of Psychology
University of California, San Diego
USA

Dr Janet Nicol
Department of Psychology
University of Arizona, Tucson
USA

Dr Maria M. Piñango
Department of Linguistics
Yale University, New Haven, CT
USA
and
Aphasia Research Center
Boston VA Medical Center
USA

Judith Rispens, MA
Department of Dutch
University of Groningen
The Netherlands

Prof Dr Lewis P. Shapiro
Department of Communication
Sciences and Disorders
San Diego State University
USA

Prof Dr David Swinney
Department of Psychology
University of California, San Diego
USA

Dr Ron von Zonneveld
Department of Dutch
University of Groningen
The Netherlands

Prof Dr Edgar B. Zurif
Volen Center for Complex Sciences
Linguistics and Cognitive Science
Brandeis University
USA
and
Aphasia Research Center
Boston VA Medical Center
USA

Introduction

ROELIEN BASTIAANSE

The present book gives an overview of the field of neurolinguistic studies at the end of the 1990s from a group of people who study the subject from the same angle. They all focus on agrammatic Broca's aphasia and they look at different aspects of the linguistic processes and at different languages. There are two central issues. The first is how healthy and aphasic speakers deal with certain syntactic operations, such as reflexives, unaccusativity and passivization. The second subject is the production of verbs in several languages (Dutch, English, Hebrew and Hungarian). Different methods of investigations have been used: cross-modal priming to assess on-line processing, picture pointing to evaluate comprehension, naming tasks to elicit verbs in isolation and in sentence context and spontaneous speech analysis. The results from these investigations yield a wide range of data that have been interpreted within a linguistic framework, more specifically in a framework of Universal Grammar (UG).

The first chapter, by Lewis Shapiro, is an introduction to this framework and a guide is given for those who are not familiar with syntactic trees, movement rules and concepts like Government and Binding. All the background information that is needed for non-linguists in order to understand the information in the other chapters is provided here.

The second chapter, again written by Lewis Shapiro, describes two experiments performed with healthy speakers, in which on-line processing of long-distance relations has been tested. The first study focuses on complex predicate-ellipses, such as *the woman asserted herself and the pilot did too*, where the missing object in the second part (which we would expect to be a pronoun) refers to *the pilot*, although syntactically speaking it could refer to *the woman* as well. On-line processing shows that non-brain-damaged listeners also reactivate the meaning of *the woman*, a constituent that could be the antecedent according to syntactic rules, but not according to verb semantics. The second experiment studies on-line processing of *wh*-questions, both *who*- and *what*-questions and *which*-questions. The latter kind are supposed to be referential (they include participants taking part in the event described, *which girl*) and discourse-linked (they pick out an individual from a group). Non-brain-damaged listeners need less time to process the non-discourse-linked question-words *who* and *what* than the discoursed-linked *which*- questions. Shapiro argues that discourse-linking requires additional processing time, because extra-syntactic information is involved. In combination with the outcomes of the first experiment, it is concluded that reactivation of an antecedent's meaning is syntactically driven and it is immediate, that is, at the original position of the antecedent. If, however, extra-syntactic information is required, the reactivation of the antecedent's meaning is delayed.

In Chapter 3, David Swinney, Tracy Love, Janet Nicol, Vikki Bouck and Lea Ann Hald focus on the correlates between neuro-anatomic organization and human language processing by studying on-line sentence processing and sentence comprehension in both non-brain-damaged and aphasic speakers. First, on-line processing and comprehension of long-distance dependencies are tested in the two subject groups. Long-distance dependencies are relations between constituents in the sentence that are broken by other constituents. This may be a co-referential relation between a pronoun and its antecedent (*the waitress told the baker that she would be late*) or between so-called 'moved' constituents and their original position, as in object-relative sentences (*the waitress$_i$ who the customer accused t$_i$ of rude behaviour*). In sentences like this, the object *the waitress* is supposed to be moved from the original object position, but a dependency-relation remains, as indicated by the index i in the example. In healthy speakers, the meaning of the antecedent (in the above examples *the waitress*) is shown to be reactivated at the position of the pronoun or the original position of the object (in the above example indicated with i), but neither earlier, nor later. A similar pattern is found for Wernicke's aphasics, but not for Broca's aphasics, suggesting that Broca's area plays an essential role in linking constituents during sentence processing. It is shown that this reactivation is not a conscious process: healthy listeners sometimes give a syntactically incorrect reading to an implausible sentence, although on-line measuring shows that the syntactic processing was done adequately.

In Chapter 4, Edgar Zurif and Maria Piñango consider the functioning of the interface between semantics and syntax in healthy speakers and aphasics. This study focuses on specific kinds of verbs, that is, verbs that may have two readings in a sentence: a transparent one and a so-called *enriched* one, that implies that the action has been performed repeatedly. Compare the following examples: *John dived into the water* versus *John dived for an hour.* An on-line processing task in healthy speakers shows that verbs that may have an enriched reading (e.g. *to dive*) take longer to process that those with verbs that do not allow an enriched reading (e.g. *to swim*). An off-line task was presented to Wernicke's and Broca's aphasics, showing that Broca's aphasics have no problems in understanding the two readings, but Wernicke's aphasics do. The authors claim that Wernicke's area is essential for processing information at the interface level between semantics and syntax.

Chapter 5, by Maria Piñango elaborates on processing at this interface level to evaluate the processing of *unaccusatives* (verbs that select arguments that have undergoer-like characteristics, such as *to fall, to bounce, to break*) and so-called *unergatives* (verbs that select arguments with agent-like properties, such as *to run, to sleep, to jump*). Piñango shows that these types of verbs have similar semantic characteristics but differ in the underlying syntactic construction in which they are used. She shows that the usual dichotomy in comprehending active and passive sentences in Broca's aphasics does not appear in sentences with unaccusative and unergative verbs. She therefore suggests that the problems that Broca's aphasics encounter with passive sentences (and other sentences in non-canonical word-order, like object relatives and object clefts) are not caused by the non-canonicity of the grammatical roles but by the non-canonicity of the thematic roles.

Chapter 6 by Jennifer Balogh and Yosef Grodzinsky, the last chapter on the receptive disorders in Broca's aphasia, is a study of the interaction between different levels of linguistic representation and the syntactic deficit. A semantic (referentiality) and a phonetic (implicitness) property of arguments have been varied. They show that there is an interaction between these properties and Theta-role assignment in the comprehension of Broca's aphasics. There is an above-chance performance in the comprehension of passives with quantified subjects and an at-chance performance on truncated passives. This is in conjunction with the standard finding of above-chance performance on actives and at-chance on agentive passives. Balogh and Grodzinsky conclude that the knowledge of information on referentiality is not only accessible to the agrammatic aphasics, but also interacts with their deficit. They also conclude that information about implicit arguments is represented in these aphasics. These results support Grodzinsky's *Trace-Based Account (TBA)* of agrammatic comprehension.

Taking the findings on the processing and comprehension studies together, one sees that syntactic information is a crucial factor in sentence processing and comprehension (as shown by Shapiro, Swinney and colleagues and Balogh and Grodzinsky), but it is not the only factor that is influential in normal language processing or compromised in Broca's aphasia. Shapiro shows that extra-syntactic information, such as discourse-linking, plays a role and Zurif and Piñango demonstrate that both in non-brain-damaged subjects and in Broca's aphasics the interface level between syntax and semantics is essential for meaning. Piñango's findings and those of Balogh and Grodzinsky are at some stage contradictory: although, according to the latter authors the comprehension deficit in

Broca's aphasia should be explained in purely syntactic terms, that is the non-canonicity of the grammatical roles, Piñango argues for a more semantically orientated account: the non-canonicity of the thematic roles. The future will tell which theory provides a better description of the comprehension disorders in Broca's aphasia.

The second part of the book is on agrammatic production and focuses on the production of verbs. In Chapter 7 Roel Jonkers presents the data of his study on the effect of transitivity on (Dutch) agrammatics' abilities to retrieve verbs from the lexicon. Lemmas of transitive verbs carry more syntactic and semantic information than intransitive verbs. Jonkers' question is whether this has an effect on accessing verbs and if so, whether this effect is the same at the word and the sentence level. He finds that his group of agrammatic patients is significantly better in retrieving transitive verbs when they have to name pictures of actions (such as: *to cut* and *to throw* versus *to swim* and *to crawl*). At the sentence level, however, this effect disappears. Analysis shows that this is strongly related to the subjects' ability to construct sentences: patients who are better in retrieving transitive than intransitive verbs at the sentence level produce more subjects and objects than patients who show the opposite pattern (better in retrieving intransitive than transitive verbs at the sentence level).

In Chapter 8, Katalin Kiss studies the role of verb complexity on sentence production of (Hungarian) agrammatic patients. Hungarian is a very interesting language in this respect, because many properties that are expressed by grammatical words in language like English (such as reflexives) are grammatical affixes of the verb in Hungarian (e.g. *vakarózik = scratch oneself, nyújtózkodik = to stretch oneself*). Kiss tested two agrammatics on a sentence-construction task. Both the morphological complexity and the required number of arguments were varied. One- and two-placed verbs were easiest to access and the representational complexity also had a direct effect on the accessibility of the predicates: the more complex the verb, the more difficult they were to retrieve. Analysis shows, however, that when the lexical form of the target verbs cannot be accessed, the correct number of arguments is realized and activation of the arguments was related to thematic hierarchy. Kiss concludes that there is an asynchronity between two mechanisms: semantic operations and syntactic processing cannot function simultaneously: sometimes the correct argument structure and thematic information is accessed and sometimes the construction of the phrase structure is correct, including mapping the arguments into the syntactic frame. Only when syntactic operations and mapping work in parallel, can a grammatical sentence be produced and this is exactly the point where the agrammatic speaker fails.

Chapter 9, by Na'ama Friedmann, is about the production of inflected verbs in agrammatic production. According to her theory, the problems with verb inflection are caused by an underlying syntactic disorder that prevents the agrammatic speakers from using finite verb forms in their proper position. Agrammatics therefore choose verb forms that are non-finite. Thus, infinitives, gerunds and participles are produced. Friedmann presents a syntactic account of this phenomenon. This allows her to predict which forms will be produced in which position in the sentence in different languages. These predictions have been tested for Hebrew, Dutch and German, among other languages. The cross-linguistic data support Friedmann's account: agrammatics cannot produce certain functional categories, because of their position in the sentence. Which categories are affected is dependent on the language of the agrammatic speaker.

In Chapter 10, Roelien Bastiaanse, Judith Rispens and Ron van Zonneveld present further, experimental data on verb inflection and related issues. In the first study, they compare the retrieval and inflection of verbs in spontaneous speech of a group of agrammatic speakers. Analysis of the individual data shows that two patterns of performance are discernible: half of the patients show a low variety in the verbs they produce, but they produce a relatively large number of inflected verbs; the other half of the group demonstrates the opposite pattern: virtually normal variety of verbs, but poor on the production of inflected verbs. The authors conclude that there is apparently a grammatical factor that influences the lexical abilities in spontaneous speech. In a second study, they show that this factor is syntactic in nature and not morphological: agrammatic speakers are able to produce finite verbs, as long as they remain in their canonical position. The last study focuses on negation, a concept related to verb finiteness in some languages (like English) but not in others (like Dutch). The data show that in agrammatic speakers of a language with a dependency relation between the finite verbs and negation, negation is more impaired than in agrammatic speakers of a language where there is no such relation. The authors therefore suggest that not only finite verbs are affected in agrammatic speech, but also other categories that are related to them.

In Chapter 11, the final chapter, Susan Edwards shows the clinical merits of the type of experimental research reported in the earlier chapters. She presents an agrammatic Broca's aphasic, who has been tested with a wide range of comprehension and production tests, both at the word and at the sentence level. Additionally several narrative samples have been analysed. The results resonate with the group research findings reported by the authors in this volume. The patient is poor in action naming, both at the word and at the sentence level, with an effect for transitivity at the word level. She has problems with the grammatical features in spontaneous speech, but there is a trade-off between the variety of grammatical structures and the variety of verbs she produces. When she produces more embedded structures, the diversity of verbs drops. The variation in distribution is exposed by comparing three different types of narratives. Such findings, it is argued, are crucial for aphasia therapy. Only when the exact nature of the underlying disorder is known, can one design a therapy programme to teach the patient how to circumvent their problems and/or to use strategies to compensate for the most prominent features of the disorder.

Taking the results given in the second part of the book, the chapters which report on production data, we can conclude that verbs make speech difficult for agrammatic speakers: retrieval of verbs from the lexicon, the realization of argument structure and inflection are all affected. Two things are important here, however. One is that there may be a striking difference between languages in the verb production of agrammatic speakers. Kiss and Jonkers find different effects for certain properties of the verbs in Hungarian and Dutch, and Friedmann shows that the degree in which verb inflection is affected is dependent on the grammar of the language the agrammatic patient speaks. The other is shown by Bastiaanse and colleagues: in spontaneous speech not each agrammatic exhibits the same weaknesses or deficits, despite the assumed same underlying disorder; some patients tend to focus on communicative content, at the cost of verb inflection, whereas others focus on finite verbs at the cost of the diversity of the verbs, a trade-off mechanism that is also noticed by Kiss. This diversity of performance can even be found within a single patient depending on the assessment protocol used, as demonstrated by Edwards.

All in all, this book gives an overview of the state of the art of the neurolinguistic approach to agrammatism at the turn of the century and examples of how such work can motivate clinical assessment and therapy. Neurolinguistic research has arisen as the direct consequence of Chomsky's development of the theory of universals of grammar, the subsequent use of such motivate a variety of research programmes. The authors in this volume have been influenced by this work and strive to make use of Chomsky's theories to describe and explain the phenomena found in agrammatic Broca's aphasia.

As said above, this is not the only way to study agrammatism but we consider that it is an extremely interesting and fruitful one. It provides us with insights into how brain damage may affect the language system in different languages. Using Universal Grammar as a descriptive frame enables the researchers to study the effects of brain damage on the underlying language system and the effect in different languages. This cross-linguistic contribution is important in a field that is dominated by the anglo-centric view of agrammatism.

Chapter 1
An introduction to syntax

LEWIS P. SHAPIRO

Introduction

Within theoretical linguistics, *syntax* is the study of the architecture of phrases, clauses and sentences. The modern roots of the study of syntax can be traced to the pioneering work of Noam Chomsky, who in 1957 wrote *Syntactic Structures*. Chomsky changed the face of linguistics by casting its domain inwardly. That is, the concern shifted from describing external language phenomena to characterizing the mental machinery that purported to explain the native speakers' knowledge of language; that concern remains today. In this summary I borrow rather heavily from Chomsky's *Government-Binding Theory* and *Principles and Parameters* (Chomsky, 1986b, 1992).[1] The proper study of (introductory) syntax could easily take up the entire body of a large text (e.g. Van Riemsdijk and Williams, 1986; Radford, 1988; Haegeman, 1992). Because this chapter is intended as a tutorial, it will emphasize constructs that will help the reader understand the general nature of syntactic theorizing without being too concerned with theory-internal issues; the chapter also emphasizes those aspects of syntactic theory that are relevant to research in normal and disordered language performance in children and adults. Leonard and Loeb (1988) previously cut a similar path in their tutorial on Government-Binding Theory. The present chapter is intended as an update to that effort as well as a more detailed examination of syntactic theory.

So far as the intended audience is concerned, this chapter is not necessarily directed towards those researchers who are familiar with theories of syntax. Rather, it is intended for the audience of researchers or students of language who may not have a current understanding of syntax or its relevance and would like an introduction. If you are a student of language, a rudimentary knowledge of syntax is essential because it is part of the basic science of language, as are theories of phonology, morphology, semantics and discourse. Also, syntactic theory forms the backbone of much of the work in normal and disordered language processing. Indeed, understanding syntax and manipulating it in principled ways is becoming more and more important to the treatment of language disorders in both children and adults.

I'd like to begin by asking the reader to keep one thing in mind during this exercise: *A theory of syntax must describe all and only all the well-formed, acceptable sentences in any given language.* If a syntactic theory not only explains the sentences that are grammatical, but also somehow allows the generation of ungrammatical sentences, then the theory may not be an accurate characterization of our linguistic knowledge. Putting it another way, our knowledge of language allows us to make judgments regarding the sentences that are acceptable and those that are not. One purpose of a theory of syntax is to describe the mental machinery that we must possess in order to make such judgments. The theory, therefore, must explain both how we know that a particular sentence is acceptable and how we know that a particular sentence is not acceptable. As a start to the construction of this theory, consider:

1. Dillon and Joelle went to the beach
2. *Dillon and Joelle put to the beach

Our intuitions about English (driven by our unconscious linguistic knowledge) allow us effortlessly to judge (1) as acceptable (i.e. grammatical, well-formed) and (2) as unacceptable (i.e. ungrammatical, ill formed –signified by an *). If you were asked why this is so, you might hypothesize that 'sentence (1) is well formed and sentence (2) is not because they have different verbs'. But such a statement doesn't really tell us anything substantial; it's just a description of the difference between the two sentences. For example, to explain the grammaticality of (1) and the ungrammaticality of (2), we would have to know something about how we acquire the lexical category of verbs, how phrasal categories are constructed out of lexical categories, how each verb picks its linguistic environment [some verbs go with some phrases and some go with other phrases, to which both (1) and (2) attest], and how this information comes together to yield knowledge of the grammatical sentences of a language. Later, the theoretical machinery that some syntacticians claim is necessary to explain the facts about (1) and (2) will be described.

Our syntactic knowledge also allows us to go beyond making judgments about whole sentences. If (1) were to be divided into two sections, where would the division occur? It is very likely that the sentence would be divided between its *subject* (*Dillon and Joelle*) and its *predicate* (*went to the beach*). Thus, a first pass at the syntactic structure of the sentence might be:

3. [[Dillon and Joelle] [went to the beach]]

Note that the outer set of brackets demarcates the entire sentence; the inner sets of brackets divide the sentence up into further parts. But why wouldn't (1) be divided into the following?:

4. *[[Dillon and] [Joelle went to the beach]] or
5. *[[Dillon and Joelle went] [to the beach]]

Sentence (1) would likely be divided as (3) and not as (4) or (5) because you have the mental capacity to know effortlessly that (3) yields well-formed parts (or *constituents*) and that (4) and (5) do not. Now take what we have called the predicate and divide it further, into two parts:

6. [[went] [to the beach]]

What we have done in (6) is to divide the predicate into a *verb* (*went*, the past tense of *go*) and a *prepositional phrase (to the beach)*. And, of course, we can further divide the prepositional phrase into a *preposition* (*to*) and its *noun phrase* object (*the beach*).

Our grammatical knowledge also allows us to make judgments about *reference*; we know that some lexical items refer to others in the same sentence or in the discourse (i.e. extra-sentential reference). For example:

7. Dillon hit himself
8. Dillon hit him

We know that *himself* must refer to Dillon in (7), yet in (8) we know that *him* cannot refer to *Dillon*.

Our syntactic knowledge also allows us to make judgments of 'sameness of meaning'. For example:

9. Dillon hit Joelle
10. Joelle was hit by Dillon

We know that although the focus may be different in (9) and (10), the basic meaning is the same.

Finally, our syntactic knowledge allows us to recognize structural ambiguities, sometimes subtle ones:

11. The mechanic fixed the car in the garage

If some thought is given to what (11) can, in principle, mean, we come to the conclusion that it can mean either something like 'it was in the garage where the mechanic fixed the car' or it can mean 'it was the car in the garage (instead of the car outside the garage) that the mechanic fixed'.

These meanings, as we shall see later, are reflected by where the prepositional phrase (*in the car*) fits into the phrasal geometry of the sentence.

It is likely the reader cannot verbalize the rules and principles that the
judgments about examples (1)–(11) were based on, basically because
knowledge of language is *tacit* or unconscious. The job of the theoretical
syntactician is to observe, hypothesize, and test what this knowledge
consists of. The *data* that linguists primarily use to develop and test their
theories come from *grammatical intuitions* of native speakers. From
these intuitions, theoretical constructs and hypotheses are developed and
placed within a theory and then tested against new observations (new
data). Based on these new data, the theory can either be accepted, revised
or rejected. And this process of data-gathering, testing, theory development, data-gathering, goes on and on. Such is the toil of any science,
including the science of language.

In this chapter, then, aspects of a particular theory of syntax will be
summarized. These include lexical and phrasal categories and how they
are put together into clauses and sentences, how words are represented in
the mental lexicon (dictionary), how lexical properties project to the
syntax, and how noun phrases (NPs) are assigned structural and semantic
information. Additionally, I will describe how sentences that are not
canonically ordered are derived and represented (in English,
Subject–Verb–Object ordering is considered canonical, or basic), how and
to what do personal and reflexive pronouns refer, and how the principles
that connect all these theoretical notions form knowledge of language.
The chapter concludes with examples of psycholinguistic and neurolinguistic efforts that show the relevance of the study of syntax to language
performance and to the treatment of language disorders.

Lexical and functional categories

Categories are theoretical constructs that linguists use to explain the fact
that some words behave differently than others. Instead of using vague
notions like 'nouns are persons, places, or things' (the word *run* can be a
noun or a verb), 'verbs refer to action' (*destruction* is an 'action,' but is
actually a noun), and 'prepositions are words referring to locations' (*La
Jolla* is a location, but is a noun), linguists have looked to phonological,
morphological, and distributional evidence to determine or rationalize
lexical categorization, or parts of speech. For example, phonologically, the
primary stress often falls on the first syllable of multisyllabic nouns (e.g.
PERmits, RECords), yet on verbs the primary stress often falls on the
second syllable (e.g. perMITS, reCORDS). Morphologically, nouns can be
pluralized (*boys, women*) and verbs cannot. Nouns and verbs can form
complex words made up of more than one morpheme, but prepositions
cannot; they are invariant. Distributionally, nouns occur in particular and
in different parts of a sentence than do verbs; thus, they cannot be substi-

tuted for each other (they are said to be in *complementary distribution*). For example, nouns can be pre-modified by adjectives (very big *boy*, pretty *woman*, etc.) yet verbs cannot (*very big *know*); nouns can be quantified and specified (e.g. made definite or indefinite) (e.g. *the boy, a boy*), yet verbs cannot (**a/the know*). So, a verb cannot be substituted for a noun, and vice versa (*Dillon kissed Joelle*, **Kissed Dillon Joelle*). Indeed, substitution is one *constituency test* that linguists use to help determine the category of a lexical item.

Because of these phonological, morphological and distributional facts, linguists have hypothesized a limited set of *lexical* categories such as Nouns, Verbs, Adjectives and Prepositions, as well as a set of *functional* categories like Determiners (*the, this, some, many* etc.), Complementizers (*that, whether, for* etc.) and Inflections (modals such as *will* and *should*, for example, and tense and agreement morphemes). Claiming that there are distinct categories that behave differently allows the linguist to make general statements, like 'nouns can be pluralized, verbs cannot'. Such general statements allow lexical items to be represented *economically*. For example, because only nouns can be pluralized, it is not necessary to represent the plural noun separately from its singular version. All that is needed is a representation of the singular noun and a *rule* that states that nouns can be pluralized; this will automatically generate the plural form for the noun. Importantly, this productive mechanism simplifies the acquisition process that the child undergoes. That is, the child does not need to 'memorize' each plural form for each singular noun counterpart; all the child needs to know is the rule for the plural and the fact that any noun can have a plural form (although the child will indeed have to memorize irregular forms). This emphasis on language acquisition forms the basis for much of linguistic theory.

Phrasal categories and phrase structures

Categories such as nouns, verbs and prepositions are not just arranged in a one-level left-to-right serial order. Instead, evidence suggests that they form *phrasal categories*, and both lexical, functional and phrasal categories are arranged in a *hierarchical structure* to form clauses and sentences, much like a house is built with a foundation, walls, beams and a roof. Again, consider the sentence *The mechanic fixed the car in the garage*. The ambiguity that was described earlier is not lexical; none of the crucial words in the sentence has more than one sense. How, then, can we account for the ambiguity?

One way to explain this phenomenon is to assume that phrases are organized into hierarchical structures and that there will be cases where more than one structure can be assigned to a particular phrase. Thus, *The mechanic fixed the car in the garage* can be assigned two different structures. The two structures can be viewed in different ways. For example, an approximation of the two structures can be viewed by different *labelled bracketing*:

12. [S [NP The mechanic] [VP fixed [NP1 [NP2 the car] [PP in the garage]]]]
13. [S [NP The mechanic] [VP fixed [NP the car] [PP in the garage]]]

In (12), the prepositional phrase (PP) *in the garage* modifies the noun phrase (NP2) *the car*; thus, there is one larger NP (NP1), *the car in the garage* (I have boldfaced the brackets in this case). In (13) the PP *in the garage* modifies the entire verb phrase (VP) *fixed the car* (later, I will rid phrasal notation of numbered nodes such as NP1 and NP2 in favour of a more parsimonious representation). Another method of showing *phrasal geometry* is through the *phrase structure tree (phrase marker)*. Examples (14) and (15) show a first-pass at the two phrase structure trees for the ambiguous sentences, (12) and (13), respectively (see Figures 1.1 and 1.2):

14.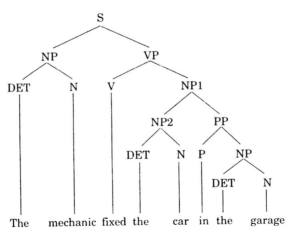

Figure 1.1

15.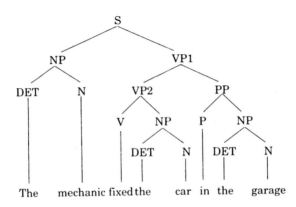

Figure 1.2

Viewing just the verb phrase (VP) for a moment, in (14) the PP *in the garage* modifies the noun phrase *the car* and thus attaches to the 'higher' NP1 node, forming an NP *the car in the garage*; in (15) the PP *in the garage* modifies the VP and thus attaches to the 'higher' VP1 node, forming the 'higher' *VP fixed the car in the garage*. So, the structure of the sentences of a language can be captured by phrase structure representations, where each structure suggests a specific interpretation.

Continuing with examples (14) and (15), consider in more detail the symbols used to label phrase structure nodes. There is a distinction between *lexical nodes* and *phrasal nodes*. Lexical nodes are made up of lexical categories such as noun (N), verb (V) and preposition (P). Phrasal nodes include phrasal categories such as noun phrases (NPs), verb phrases (VPs), and prepositional phrases (PPs). For example, the sentence *the mechanic ate* contains a noun phrase (NP) *the mechanic*, which in turn contains the noun (N) *mechanic*. Phrase structure theory contains a principle that captures an important generalization about the structure of these categories:

16. The Head Principle: Every phrasal category contains a head; the head and its phrasal counterparts share the same properties.

An NP must contain an N, which is the *head* of the NP, a VP must contain a V, and so on; the head and its phrase share properties. For example, if a head noun is plural, so too is the entire NP (e.g. *The boys* are wild). This principle serves as an important constraint on phrase structure representations; if there were no such constraint, phrase structures would allow the generation of impossible structures (e.g. an NP containing a V).

Continuing, an analysis of English sentences tells us that a sentence consists of both a noun phrase and a predicate (i.e. a verb phrase). Example (17) is a shorthand way of stating this property:

17. S → NP VP: [S [NP The mechanic] [VP fixed the car in the garage]]

The arrow, for now, means 'is rewritten as' or 'consists of', so (17) says that an S can be rewritten as an NP and a VP. An NP, in turn, consists of a noun (obligatory), which may or may not be preceded by a determiner (optionality is denoted by a set of parentheses), as in:

18. NP → (DET) N: [NP [DET The] [N mechanic]]

A verb phrase consists of at least a verb, and potentially many other optional elements, including another NP, a PP, or even another Sentence (clause). (Examples of some of these possibilities are shown in (19):

19. VP → V: [VP [V slept]]

```
V NP:        [VP [V fixed] [NP the car]]
V NP PP:     [VP [V sent] [NP the letter] [PP to his mother]]
V S:         [VP [V discovered] [S that the manuscript was stolen]]
```

A prepositional phrase may include a preposition followed by an NP, as in:

20. PP → P NP: [PP [P in] [NP the garage]]

Finally, there is one important constraint on phrase structures that has been left out. Consider:

21. S → NP VP
    VP → V NP

To generate a sentence given a particular set of phrase structures, lexical items are inserted into the category slots via *lexical insertion*. A grammatical sentence corresponding to (21) might be:

22. Joelle *kicked* the door,

where *Joelle* is lexically inserted into the N slot of the subject NP, *kick* into the V slot of the VP, and *the door* into the direct object NP. But what about the following?:

23. *Joelle *thinks* the door

Sentence (23) has the same structure as (22), can fit into the phrase structure representation described in (21), and yet our intuitions tell us that it is not a well-formed sentence in English. What makes (22) different from (23)? The only difference lexically between the two sentences is, of course, the verb. If the verb *kick* is inserted in the phrase structure of (21), the sentence is well-formed; if the verb *think* is inserted, the sentence is ill-formed. So, the theory of grammar as it stands now is simply too powerful; it generates ungrammatical as well as grammatical sentences. The theory, therefore, must have a way to restrict the output of phrase structure representations like those in (21) to *generate only the well-formed instances of our language*. Before this problem is tackled, some generalizations about phrase structures that have given rise to what is called *X-bar Theory* need to be detailed.

X-bar Theory

X-bar Theory is a formal way of characterizing what is common about phrase structures. Recall that each phrasal category must contain a head (16). For NPs, the head is the N, for VPs, the V, and so on. But what could be the head of the S-node in, for example, (14) and (15)? To answer this question, note that sentences have *inflection*; they are inflected for tense (TNS) and agreement (AGR). At first it might appear that it is not the sentence that has tense, but, instead, the VP. For example, in the sentence, *The mechanic fixed the car in the garage*, it appears that the VP is past tense, because the head of the VP (the V) has past tense morphology (*-ed*). But consider that the past tense can be separated from the VP, as in *What the mechanic did was fix the car*, where the past tense is now part of the auxiliary *did* and is no longer 'attached' to the verb itself. Also consider that overt, non-affix tense markers like *will*, for example (e.g. *The mechanic will fix the car*), are separated from the VP. For these and other reasons, linguists now consider tense to be represented separately from the verb and verb phrase, forming what is called an inflection phrase (IP). The head of IP is the functional category INFL or I (for inflection).

Consider again (14), repeated in (24), but this time with a more fully specified phrasal architecture (see Figure 1.3):

24.

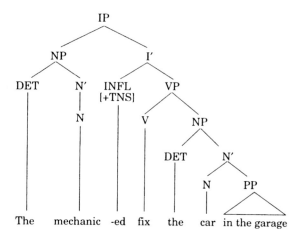

Figure 1.3

First, note the following terms: *branching* means that a node splits into other nodes, *dominates* means that a given node is 'higher up in the tree' than other nodes, and *immediately dominates* means that a given node is directly above another node in the tree, with no other nodes intervening between them. In (24), the S-node is now replaced by an IP that dominates all other nodes of the tree. The IP branches and immediately dominates an NP and an intermediate structure (called I-bar; written as I') whose head is INFL (which, in this case, is past tense). The subject NP branches and immediately dominates DET (determiner) and an intermediate category, N'. N' immediately dominates the head N. The I' also has a VP attached 'to the right'. This schema thus retains the generalization that all phrases must have a head although accepting our intuitions that sentences have inflections that are independent from verbs and verb phrases.

Example (24) has several other generalizations. Note that the V has as its *complement* an NP (*the car in the garage*). And note that the head V (*fix*) falls 'to the left' of its complement. If we were to draw out the PP, we would also note that the head P (*in*) also falls to the left of its NP complement *the garage*. The same holds true for the INFL node (*-ed*), which falls to the left of its complement, the VP (*fix the car in the garage*). So it seems that one generalization about (24) – and indeed all phrase structure (PS) rules of English – is that the head occurs to the *left* of its complements. This particular order of heads and their complements is not a universal property of all languages; languages generally fall into two camps, *head-first* or *head-last*.[2]

Another generalization is that the determiner modifies or *specifies* the NP; the NP can be definite, indefinite, quantified, personalized and so forth. So, for example, we could have *a mechanic, the mechanic, some mechanic, all mechanics*, and so forth. We will assume that the subject NP inhabits a functional category position called Spec (for Specifier); I will continue, however, to fill this Spec position with an NP.

Note that instead of using node labels like NP1 and NP2, I am now using XP and X' (where XP stands for NP, VP, PP etc.). This X-bar notation captures the generalization that all phrase structure representations have the same form.[3,4]

Consider now the structure of *clauses*:

25. Joelle wondered whether the boy ate

The lexical item *whether* is a Complementizer (as are *that, if* and *for* in English) that often signals an embedded clause. Because each phrasal type has a head that shares the properties of the phrase, the Complementizer *whether* heads a complementizer phrase (a CP). Given these assumptions, consider the approximate structure of (25), shown in (26):

In (26), the verb *wonder* appears in the *matrix clause* (the topmost or main clause) and the verb *eat* appears in the *embedded clause*. The IP dominates all nodes and branches immediately to dominate an NP and an I'. The subject NP immediately dominates an N', which immediately dominates an N (*Joelle*). The I' branches immediately to dominate its head, the INFL node, and the VP. The VP immediately dominates a V', which branches and immediately dominates its head V (*wonder*) and an embedded CP (*whether the boy ate*), which is the complement (argument) of the V. The CP, in turn, branches to a Specifier position

26.

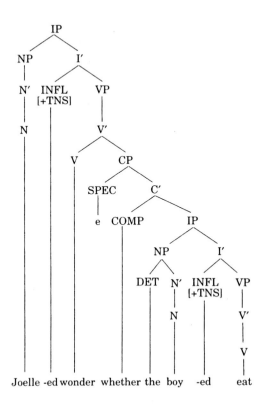

Figure 1.4

(which is empty; more on this later) and to a C'. The C' branches and immediately dominates its head Complementizer (COMP) (*whether*) and an IP (*the boy eat*). The IP branches and immediately dominates the DET position (*the*) and an NP. The NP branches and immediately dominates an N' (which dominates the N) and an I', which branches and immediately dominates its head INFL node (+TNS) and a VP The VP immediately dominates a V', which dominates its head V (*eat*).

To simplify matters a bit, consider the following generalizations shown in (27) and (28):

27. All phrase structures have the same form: an XP (maximal projection), X'(s) (intermediate projections), a head X (a lexical category), a complement (ZP) of the head that is on the same phrasal level as the head, a Specifier position, and, perhaps, an adjunct phrase (modifier; YP) that can attach above the head.

28. X-bar schema:

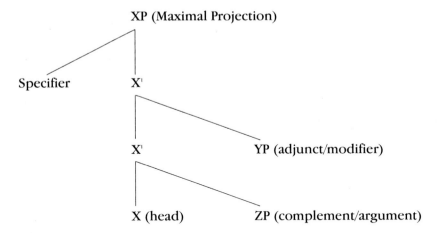

Figure 1.5

According to (28) the head (X, sometimes referred to as X^0) is an atomic element (a category) drawn from the lexicon. Phrase markers are *projected* from the head to intermediate levels (e.g. N', V', etc.) and to a maximal projection (e.g. NP, VP etc.). The *complement* of the head is often called its *argument*, which is syntactically on the same phrasal level as the head (the head and its arguments are therefore said to be 'sisters'). The *specifier* is immediately dominated by the maximal projection and is a sister to the X' level, and the *adjunct* is often immediately dominated by an intermediate projection. Importantly, the terms *specifier*, *argument* and *adjunct* are not formal category terms (like NP, N', etc.) but are, instead, relational terms so that we speak of the *argument of X, the specifier of XP* and so on. For example, a subject NP is the specifier of IP, a direct object NP is an argument of the verb, and so forth.

This schema and the trees depicted in (14), (15), (24) and (26) assume *binary branching* (Kayne, 1984), whereby an X-bar category can at most immediately dominate two nodes. One reason behind constraining trees to binary branching has to do with learnability. It could be argued that if the binary branching constraint is part of a child's tacit knowledge of language, then fewer decisions will need to be made regarding the structure of the language. Hence, acquiring a language will be 'faster' and 'less effortful' than if the grammar allowed unconstrained branching.

Because all phrase structures conform to the X-bar schema in (28), the acquisition of the phrasal geometry of sentences becomes a matter of acquiring *the order* in which the specifier, head and adjuncts fall. According to the Principles and Parameters approach, children have, as part of their innate capacity to acquire language, knowledge of this X-bar schema. There is also a limited set of parameters that must be set via experience in their native language, parameters, for example, that allow children to order these constituents. As will be evident shortly, acquiring the lexicon (i.e. mental dictionary) of the language makes this task easier.

Structural relations

Consider now two important formal relations among the nodes of a tree; the first of these is known as *c-command*:

29. A node X c-commands a node Y if and only if the first branching node dominating X also dominates Y.

Using (26) as an example, the subject NP c-commands I' (and vice versa) because the first branching node dominating the NP is IP, which also dominates I'. The V c-commands CP (the verb's complement or argument) because the first branching node dominating V is V', which also dominates CP.

The fact that *heads c-command their arguments* sets the stage for another local relation, known as *Government*:

30. A node X *governs* a node Y if and only if

(a) X c-commands Y,
(b) X and Y are in the same (maximal) projection, and
(c) no maximal projection intervenes between X and Y

On most versions of Government the *governor* must be a head (either a functional or lexical category). Using (26) once again as an example, a head (e.g. V) governs its internal argument(s) (e.g. CP in the matrix clause); that is, V c-commands CP, V and CP are in the same maximal projection (VP), there are no intervening maximal projections between V and CP, and V the governor of CP is a lexical category.

It turns out that the principle of Government yields several other principles, including subcategorization, thematic role assignment, case assignment and trace–antecedent relations. These will be discussed in the following sections.

The Lexicon and Theta Theory

Before describing X-bar syntax, the point was made that phrase structure rules, by themselves, are too powerful; that is, their output can generate both grammatical and ungrammatical sentences. Again, because – at this point in our theorizing – lexical insertion can pull out any verb to fill the V-node, some sentences will turn out to be grammatical (e.g. 'Joelle *kicked* the door') and some will turn out ungrammatical ('Joelle *thinks* the door'). One way for the theory to constrain or to restrict the output of phrase structures to allow only well-formed sentences is through information represented in the *Mental Lexicon* or mental dictionary. The Lexicon contains representations of the list of words of a language that a speaker has acquired and stored in memory. Included in each word's lexical entry is information about its phonological form (how it is spoken or read), its lexical category (verb, noun, preposition etc.), semantic information (what it refers to in the real world), and importantly, the legal sentence environments the word is allowed to enter. As was shown above, for example, not all words, in this case verbs, can fit into all types of sentence structures.

It will turn out that verbs are crucial to accounts of syntactic representation as well as to accounts of sentence processing. Each verb carries two types of syntactic well-formedness information: *strict subcategorization* and *argument structure*; argument structure, in turn, interacts with the more semantic notion of *thematic roles*.

Subcategorization

By subcategorization we mean the type of syntactic environment into which a verb can enter. In particular, it is a characterization of the *type of phrasal category* that follows the verb (in head-first languages). Consider the following two examples:

31. [NP Dillon] [VP [V kissed] [NP Joelle]]
32. [NP Dillon] [VP [V put [NP the toy] [PP on the shelf]]

The verb *kiss* requires a direct object NP (*Joelle*) and the verb *put* requires both an NP (*the toy*) and a PP (*on the shelf*). Thus, *kiss* is said to subcategorize for an NP, and *put* for an NP PP. The fact that our knowledge of English tells us that *kiss* must be followed by an NP renders the sentence **Joelle kissed* incomplete, or ungrammatical; the subcategorization for *kiss* is not satisfied in this sentence. Verbs in principle can subcategorize for any phrase type, or combinations of phrases, but each verb chooses its allowable phrasal environment.

Such information is represented as part of the verb's entry in the lexicon. Partial entries for *hit* and *put*, for example, would be:

33. *kiss* V (lexical category)
    /kIs/ (phonology)
    [_NP] (subcategorization)

34. *put* V (lexical category)
    /put/ (phonology)
    [_NP PP] (subcategorization)

As shown in (33) and (34), information in the lexicon (i.e. subcategorization information) restricts the output of the phrase structure rules of a grammar to only well-formed instances of a language. That is, if it is assumed that the subcategorization frame for each verb must be satisfied in the sentence in which the verb is contained, then we ensure that the correct verb will be inserted in its proper structural configuration. Again, if the phrase structure allows the generation of a sentence like 'Joelle___the door', only a verb that allows a direct object NP can be inserted in the (blank) verb slot.

Indeed, there is a principle that formally describes this constraint on well-formedness:

35. The Projection Principle: Lexical representations (e.g. subcategorization possibilities) are projected to the syntax.

Given the lexical representations in (33) and (34), *Dillon kiss and *Dillon put on the shelf are ruled out by the Projection Principle because the subcategorization frame for each verb does not project to the syntax. That is, the verb kiss requires a direct object NP, and it is missing in the sentence Dillon kiss; the verb put requires both an NP and a PP, and the NP, again, is missing from Dillon put on the shelf. This principle is quite powerful and rationalizes syntax in the following sense: *When we acquire a lexical item, we acquire facts about the item's syntactic privileges of occurrence.*

As shown in (26) with wonder, verbs can also subcategorize for sentential clauses:

36. [NP Joelle] knew [NP the answer]
37. [NP Joelle] knew [CP that the answer was correct]

(36) and (37) show that the verb know selects either a direct object NP or a sentential clause (CP), and thus would have the following (abbreviated) lexical entry:

38. *know* V
    /no/
    [_NP
    CP]

It turns out that for a verb to subcategorize for a particular complement, it must *govern* that complement. For example, in (26) the matrix V wonder governs its complement, the CP *whether the boy ate.*

Argument structure

Most sentences can be considered representations of relations between a predicate and its arguments, hence the term *argument structure*. An NP or a CP can be an argument of a verb if it occupies what is called an *argument position* (i.e. subject and complement positions). Unlike subcategorization information, argument structure is not concerned with the syntactic form of the phrasal categories a verb allows, but instead is concerned with the number of participants described by the verb. The transitive verb kiss requires two participants, a 'kisser' and a 'kissee'; thus, it selects for two arguments and hence a *two-place* argument structure. The verb put requires three participants and thus entails a *three-place* argument structure. Arguments and argument structures are often represented as variables (x, y and z):

39. [Dillon x] [VP kissed [Joelle y]]
40. [Dillon x] [VP put [the ball y] on [the shelf z]]

Note that in (39) one of the arguments (y) falls within the bracketed domain of the VP, and in (40) two of the arguments (y and z) also fall within the VP. These arguments are often called *internal* because they fall within the internal configuration of the VP; the subject argument (x) is often called *external* because it falls outside the maximal projection of the verb phrase.

The verb *know* also allows a two-place argument structure, although the arguments can have different syntactic realizations:

41. [Joelle x] [VP knew [NP the answer y]]
42. [Joelle x] [VP knew [CP that the answer was correct y]]

In (41) the internal, y-argument has a different semantic status than does the internal, y-argument in (42), although the verb is the same. Roughly, in (41) the argument is the Theme of 'knowing' whereas in (42) the argument is an Event or Proposition. Thus, arguments have different syntactic as well as semantic roles to play in the sentence; these 'semantic' roles are discussed in the next section.

Thematic and semantic roles

Consider the following sentences:

43. Joelle melted *the wax*.
44. *The wax* melted.

First, notice that the NP (*the wax*) appears to play the object role of the verb *melted* in (43), yet plays a subject role of *melted* in (44). Secondly, notice that although the NPs in the two sentences each serve a different role to the verb, they nevertheless seem to have something in common: the NP in both cases reflects an entity undergoing some sort of transformation ('melting'). In a sense, then, the NP seems to be playing a *similar* role in both sentences. Consider also:

45. *The wax* was melted by *Joelle*
46. It was *Joelle* who melted *the wax*
47. It was *the wax* that was melted by *Joelle*

Although the arguments of the verb *melted* (*Joelle, the wax*) occur in different positions in (45)–(47), they also seem to play a similar role. In each case *Joelle* appears to be the *Agent* of the melting, and in each case *the wax* appears to be the *Theme* of the melting. The generalization that arguments can play similar roles although appearing in different syntactic positions rationalizes, in part, the notion of *thematic roles*, which are thematic-semantic notions of the sort that answers the question 'who did what to whom?' Each argument, then, takes on a certain thematic role (e.g. Agent, Experiencer, Theme, Patient, Goal, Benefactive etc.). Each verb selects sets of thematic roles assigned to its arguments; each set of roles is called a *thematic grid*. Like both subcategorization and argument structure, thematic properties are written into the representation of the head (e.g. the Verb) as part of the lexical entry.

Thematic roles are *assigned* to arguments in the sentence, usually by the head, which has the property of being a *Theta-assigner*. Theta-assigners are typically the lexical categories of verb, preposition, noun and adjective (in contrast to functional categories, which are not Theta-assigners). For example, the verb *kiss* requires a two-place argument structure (x y) and assigns to each argument a thematic role taken from its thematic grid; the preposition *in* is also a Theta-assigner:

48. *kiss*   V   *in*   P
             (Agent Patient)   (Location)

[Dillon AGENT] kissed [Joelle PATIENT] [in [the park LOCATION]

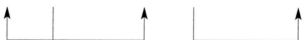

As (48) shows, the verb *kiss* assigns its thematic roles of Agent and Patient to the subject and direct-object positions, respectively (technically, the Agent role is assigned by the VP, that is, the entire VP. Of course, the properties of the VP depend on the properties of the head V, so for present purposes we will assume that the V assigns a role to the external as well as internal arguments). *Theta Theory* states that the predicate assigns its associated thematic roles to particular grammatical positions. A transitive verb like *kiss* will have two thematic roles to assign, one associated with the subject position and one associated with the object position [in the Principles and Parameters approach, object position is internal to the VP, whereas subject position falls outside the VP (but see note 4)]. Within the PP (*in the park*), the preposition *in* is the head of the PP and assigns the role of Location to its argument (*the park*).

Two important principles constrain assignment of thematic roles in the syntax: the Projection Principle (16) and the *Theta Criterion*:

49. Theta Criterion: Every argument (e.g. NP) in a sentence must receive one and only one thematic role; each thematic role associated with a Theta-assigner must be assigned to one and only one argument.

The Theta Criterion, much like the Projection Principle, ensures that a verb's (and a preposition's) thematic properties specified in a lexical entry will be assigned one-to-one to the arguments represented in the syntax. The syntax of a sentence, then, is determined to a large extent by the lexical properties of the head of each phrase. For example, if the verb requires one argument, only that argument should be observed in the sentence. If a verb requires two arguments, both arguments must be observed; and the same holds for three argument verbs.[5] Importantly, then, the Projection Principle can now be revised to include not only subcategorization information, but, crucially, argument structure and thematic information as well. Because the verb *kiss*, for example, requires a two-place argument structure, the thematic roles written into the verb's thematic grid must be 'projected' to the syntax.

Lexical contrasts

There are numerous *lexical alternations* that interact with the syntax in interesting ways, showing, again, how lexical properties project to the syntax. One of the most well known of these contrasts is *spray/load*:

50 a. Dillon sprayed Jello on the wall
    b. Dillon sprayed the wall with Jello

51 a. Dillon loaded the blocks on the truck
    b. Dillon loaded the truck with blocks

The verbs in (50) and (51) are said to *alternate*. In (50a) the direct object (the Theme) is *Jello* whereas the object of the preposition (serving the role of Location) is *the walls*. Yet, in (50b) the order is reversed; the location alternates syntactic positions with the object of the verb. There is also a subtle semantic difference between the (a) and (b) versions. When the object of the preposition does not express the location [as in (b)], the sentence has the sense that the *entire* wall was sprayed; this is often called the *holistic* interpretation. When the location argument is signalled by the object of the preposition [as in (a)], it has a *partitive* interpretation. This same semantic distinction holds true for the examples in (51). The semantic properties of the verb, then, translate to distinct syntactic forms.

Another well-studied example is the causative. Consider the verb *melted* again:

52 a. Joelle melted the wax
    b. The wax melted

In (52a) the verb is used as a *transitive* (that is, with a direct object) and in (52b), as an *intransitive*. In the transitive use the subject causes the action described by the verb. In the intransitive use the verb describes a *state*.

Note that these semantic properties of the verb translate to different syntactic forms.

There are many of these alternations found in language, and their existence suggests that a verb's argument structure is determined, to a large extent, by its meaning. Indeed, without getting into the details here, this work suggests that theoretical notions like thematic roles might be better explained by reference to a theory of *lexical-conceptual structure* (LCS); that is, to a theory of semantics (see, for example, Jackendoff, 1990b; for more on lexical contrasts, see Levin, 1993; for more on argument structure, see Grimshaw, 1990). A theory of LCS would claim that thematic roles like Agent, Patient, and so on, are descriptive simplifications for another level of representation. We now move out of the Lexicon and examine further how lexical properties interact with the syntax.

Trace Theory and Move-alpha

Consider now the following sentences, and how they fit into the theory thus far:

53. Dillon kissed Joelle (active)
54. Joelle was kissed ____ by Dillon (passive)
55. It was Joelle who Dillon kissed ____ ? (object cleft)
56. Who did Dillon kiss ? ____ (*wh*-question)

Despite appearing in different grammatical positions, *Dillon* seems to be the Agent and *Joelle* seems to be the Patient in (53)–(56) [in (56), *Joelle* is replaced by the NP *Who*]. The Projection Principle and the lexical entry for *kiss* require that *kiss* have a direct-object argument position to which the Patient role can be assigned. And the Theta Criterion requires that each argument position be assigned a thematic role represented in the verb's thematic grid. But it appears that (54)–(56) should be ruled out (ruled as ungrammatical) by both principles because there doesn't seem to be a direct-object position, as shown by the 'gap' (__). Our intuitions, however, tell us that these sentences are grammatical. But, how can they be grammatical if there doesn't seem to be an argument position to which to assign the Patient role?

One possibility is that there is, indeed, a direct-object position to which the role of Patient is assigned, and this position is just in the place where we expect it to be, immediately after the verb. According to the theory under consideration, it turns out that there is such a position in (54)–(56), just as there is in (53). However, in the former the positions are said to be *lexically unfilled* (or 'empty').

Assume that the direct object (*Joelle* in the examples above) originates in the canonical post-verb direct-object position and moves to a pre-verb position. The Projection Principle ensures proper thematic role assignment by requiring insertion of an *empty category* or *trace* into the position from which the category has moved. A trace is like a 'ghost' that is left behind when the NP moves; it is a lexically unfilled position acting as a 'place-holder'. The trace is then linked or *co-indexed* with the moved category, forming a *co-reference* relation between the two positions. The thematic role – in this case, the Patient – is assigned to the (original, direct-object) position occupied by the trace, and the moved category, called the *antecedent* to the trace, inherits the thematic role. Specifically, the trace of the movement and the NP that moved form a *chain*. Briefly, a chain *may* consist of two or more members that are co-indexed; each chain is considered a single argument [there are one-member chains as well, those NPs that do not co-refer with anything, like the NP *Dillon* in (53)–(56)]. The Theta Criterion can now be revised to include chains:

57. Theta Criterion: Thematic roles in a lexical entry are assigned to chains, and each chain receives one and only one thematic role.

All this brings us to, arguably, the most important insight of the Principles and Parameters theory (born from Chomsky's original work in the 1950s and 1960s; see Chomsky, 1957, 1965): there are, at this point in the discussion, (at least) two levels of representation for the sentence. The syntactic structure that exists before the NP is moved is known as the *underlying* or *d-structure* and that which exists after the NP is moved is the *s-structure*;[6] the syntactic operation that moves the NP is known technically as the *transformation Move-alpha*. An approximation of the underlying structure for the *wh*-question (56) 'Who did Dillon kiss?' is shown in (58a), and the s-structure for the sentence is shown in (58b):

58. a. Dillon did kiss [who]? – Underlying form (d-structure)

        [Did Dillon kiss [who]? – Subject-aux inversion (head-to-head movement)]

58. b. [Who]$_i$ did Dillon kiss [trace]$_i$? – s-structure

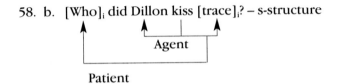

In the d-structure shown in (58a), the direct-object position is filled by the *wh*-word *who*. After *who* moves to the front of the sentence via move-alpha, it leaves behind a trace with which it is co-indexed. Note now that in the s-structure, there is a direct-object position to receive the role of Patient, although it is now occupied by the trace (i.e. it is lexically unfilled). Also, note that the thematic role of Patient is assigned to the trace position at s-structure, and the role is inherited by the moved *wh*-word *who* because the trace and its moved *wh*-phrase co-refer and form a Theta-chain. Thus, the lexical properties of the verb *kiss*, the Theta Criterion, and the Projection Principle are now satisfied.

Sentences (54) and (55) receive a similar analysis, as shown by the abbreviated s-structures in (59) and (60):

59. [Joelle]$_i$ was kissed [trace]$_i$ by Dillon
60. It was [Joelle]$_i$ [who]$_i$ Dillon kissed [trace]$_i$

Again, the lexical properties of the verb *kiss* require two arguments that are assigned the roles of Agent and Patient from its thematic grid, and there are now two positions to which the thematic roles can be assigned: the subject position that is lexically filled by the NP *Dillon*, and the direct-object position that is filled by an empty category, the trace. In (59), the direct object NP (*Joelle*) has been moved out of its canonical (i.e. 'basic') post-verb position to a position at the 'front' of the sentence, leaving behind a trace of that movement. The trace and its antecedent co-refer, and thus form a Theta-chain that is assigned the Patient role by the verb. In (60) *who* has moved from its post-verb position to a pre-verb position. The trace, *who*, and *Joelle* are co-indexed (i.e. they all co-refer) and thus form a Theta-chain; the chain is assigned the Patient role.

Another theoretical distinction is observed when the passive construction is compared to *wh*-constructions (*wh*-questions and relative clause structures). These two constructions are distinguished by what has been called *NP-movement* and *Wh-movement*, respectively (both movement types are subsumed under the general rule Move-alpha). Such a distinction has to do with, among other things, what has been called the *landing site* of the moved constituent, or the position to which a constituent moves. NP-movement involves moving an NP to an argument position (*A-position*). An A-position, again, is a position that can receive a thematic role by a Theta-assigning lexical category (a head). Typical A-positions in English include, again, the subject, direct object and indirect object (object-of-preposition). *Wh*-movement involves moving a constituent to a non-argument position (called an *A-bar position*; where 'bar' has the meaning of 'null'), a position that does not receive a thematic role and is typically a functional category such as the Specifier position. To see the difference, first consider the partial d-structure (i.e. underlying form) for the passive *Joelle was kissed by Dillon*

In (61), the direct object NP *Joelle* originates in the post-verb argument position and moves to the subject position of the sentence, occupied by an empty NP position (e) immediately dominated by the IP (we will rationalize this movement in a later section). *The NP is in an argument position* (more specifically, it is the external argument of the verb and thus

61.

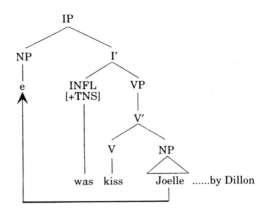

Figure 1.6

serves the role of Subject). When the direct object moves, it leaves behind a trace that is then co-indexed with the NP (the position to which it moves). The verb *kiss*, as a Theta-assigner and head, assigns the Patient role to the chain consisting of the trace and the moved NP (*Joelle*). Omitting some details here, the preposition *by*, also a lexical category and Theta-assigner, assigns the role of Agent to the NP *Dillon*.

Now consider once again the underlying form or d-structure for the *wh*-construction *Who did Dillon kiss?*, this time in terms of its phrase structure representation.

In (62), the post-verb NP (*wh*-morpheme) *who* moves to the empty (e) Specifier position, which is an A-bar position that does not receive a thematic role. Additionally, there is a second movement in (62), whereby INFL 'raises' to COMP (i.e. *did* moves to COMP). This is called head-to-head movement because the head of one phrasal type (INFL) moves to the head of another phrasal type (COMP); this used to be called Subject-to-

62.

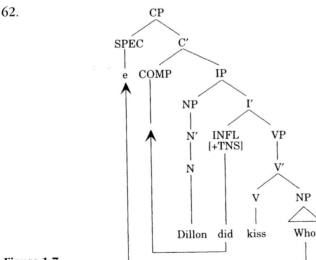

Figure 1.7

Aux inversion, explaining how, for example, *Will John go?* is derived from *John will go*. To review, then, NP-movement has an argument position landing site, yet *wh*-movement has a non-argument position landing site. Both types of movement leave behind a trace that is co-indexed with the position to which the constituent moves, and both form a chain whereby the moved constituent inherits the thematic role assigned to the internal argument position by the verb.

The Empty Category Principle (ECP)

Consider the following constraint on NP- and *wh*-traces:

63. The Empty Category Principle (ECP): A trace must be *properly governed*.

X properly governs Y if and only if

(a) X governs Y (see (31), and
(b) X is a lexical category (so that X Theta-assigns Y), or
(c) X and Y are co-indexed.

Using (62) as an example, the trace (in the direct-object position, after *who* has moved to Spec of CP) is properly governed by V because V both governs the trace (it c-commands it and is in the same maximal projection as the V) and assigns a Theta-role to the position occupied by the trace.

There are, then, two kinds of empty categories that have been described thus far: *wh*-traces and NP-traces. There is another empty category that shares some of the same properties of traces. Consider that clauses can be either finite, as in 'Joelle wondered whether the boy ate', wherein both the matrix and embedded clauses INFL is marked [+TNS] [refer back to (26)], or non-finite. The subject of a non-finite clause is an empty category called PRO (or 'big PRO'):

64. Joelle$_i$ wondered [whether [PRO]$_i$ to go home]

Although the matrix clause is finite and INFL is marked as [+TNS] (i.e. 'Joelle wondered'), the embedded clause containing the infinitive *to go* is [–TNS]. The subjects of the matrix clause (*Joelle*) and embedded clause (PRO) are said to co-refer in much the same way as was shown with traces and their antecedents.

Case Theory

Case Theory, another component of our grammar, accounts for the distribution of NPs. Consequently, it also has important implications for movement of NPs in non-canonical constructions (e.g. the passive). Case

Theory was borne out of the traditional notion of case, whereby NPs and pronouns can be distinguished by, for example, accusative, nominative, and genitive *morphological* case. Modern English has an impoverished morphological case system compared to many other languages; now only pronouns retain case in the traditional sense, and not full NPs. For example, in the sentence *He gave his car to him*, *he* is nominative, *his* is genitive, and *him* is accusative. However, what the theory is concerned with here is *not* this traditional notion of case, but, instead, a more technical notion whereby each NP must be assigned *structural* Case. Consider, then, the following principle:

65. Case Filter: *NP if NP has phonetic content and no Case.

The Case Filter means that a sentence is ungrammatical if it contains a phonetically realized NP (an NP that is 'sounded out' as opposed to an empty category) that is not assigned Case.
     Here is a very brief summary of Case Theory:

• Verbs and prepositions assign Accusative Case to their complements (arguments).
• If a clause is finite ([+TNS]), then Nominative Case is assigned to the subject NP by I (INFL). Note that the Case Filter (65) says nothing about the subject of non-finite clauses (e.g. 'Joelle wondered [whether PRO to go home]') because the subject of the clause is PRO, which does not have phonetic content and therefore is *invisible* to the Case Filter.
• Case is typically assigned under Government

Examining Case Theory further, by example, consider:

66. Joelle thought Dillon kissed Chester on the mouth

The matrix verb *think* is tensed (i.e. [+TNS]), thus INFL Case-marks the subject (*Joelle*), assigning to it Nominative Case. The embedded verb *kiss* is also tensed; thus, the embedded INFL assigns Nominative Case to the embedded subject (*Dillon*). The embedded verb *kiss* assigns Accusative Case to its object (*Chester*). The preposition *on* assigns Accusative Case to its object (*the mouth*). In each of these, the Case-assigner is a governor to its assignee.
     Consider now how the Case Filter interacts with movement and many of the other principles that have been described thus far to yield the passive.

67. The toy was given _____ to Dillon (by Joelle)
      give (Agent Theme Goal)

In (67), the direct object NP (*the toy*) has moved from its post-verb position to the front of the sentence (via NP-movement), leaving behind a trace. Note that the verb *give* has a set of thematic roles to assign, that the Projection Principle (35) states that lexical properties must be observed in the syntax and that the Theta Criterion (49) requires that all arguments must receive a thematic role and all thematic roles in a Theta-grid must be discharged. Given these principles, why is it that (67) is not ill-formed by our theory? That is, if there is no external argument in the truncated passive of (67) that can receive the role of Agent, how is the Theta Criterion satisfied? It turns out that the passive morphology (*-en*) associated with the verb has several consequences, one of which is that the Agent role is *absorbed*. The verb assigns the Theme role to the chain consisting of the moved NP (*the toy*) and its trace. The Goal is assigned to the indirect object NP (*Dillon*), and the Agent role is absorbed by the passive *-en*, allowing all three thematic roles to be discharged and thus satisfying the Theta Criterion. In the full passive version of (67), Agent cannot be assigned to the external argument (*Joelle*) because the passive morphology has absorbed this role (Agent is then assigned by the by-phrase to the external argument).

Like Theta-role absorption, another property of the passive morphology is to absorb Case. *Give* is the Case-assigner to its complement (*the toy*) yet the passive morphology takes away the ability of *give* to assign structural Case. This leaves the NP without Case, suggesting that the Case Filter will intervene and rule (67) as ill formed. To circumvent a violation of the Case Filter, *the direct object NP must move*. Movement is to subject position, where Nominative Case can then be assigned by finite INFL. In an important sense, then, Case Theory requires movement of the NP in the passive construction.

There are several commonalties between Case and Theta Theories. Both Case and Thematic roles are assigned under Government. Many Case-assigners are also Theta-assigners; many Case-assignees are also Theta-assignees. Passive morphology absorbs both Case and Theta-roles. Without getting into the details here, it turns out that many of the properties of Case Theory can indeed be derived from the properties of Theta Theory, thus simplifying the task that children have in acquiring the facts that both theories entail.

Binding Theory

Recall from the beginning of this chapter that our grammatical intuitions allow us to recognize that some lexical items co-refer and some do not:

68. Dillon hit himself
69. Dillon hit him

In (68), the lexical item in the direct-object argument position (*himself*) refers back to the subject NP argument *Dillon*. In (69), however, the direct-object argument *him* does not refer back to the subject NP. Thus, English allows two types of pronouns, a *reflexive pronoun* (or *anaphor*) shown in (68), and a *personal pronoun* (or *pronominal*) shown in (69). What generalization can be discovered about these two pronouns? First, consider that each of these constructions contains only a single clause. Next, notice that the reflexive pronoun appears to co-refer with an NP within that clause; such a relation between the two positions is called *co-reference*. The personal pronoun, on the other hand, does *not* co-refer with an NP within the clause. Given such a generalization about the two types of pronouns, consider constructions with two clauses (note that we are using *co-indexation* to describe the relation between anaphors/ pronominals and their antecedents):

70. [Rico knows] [CP that Scott$_i$ hit himself$_i$]
71. * [Rico$_i$ knows] [CP that Scott hit himself$_i$]
72. [Rico$_i$ knows] [CP that Scott hit him$_i$]
73. * [Rico knows] [CP that Scott$_i$ hit him$_i$]
74. [Rico knows] [CP that Scott hit Lola]

Does the generalization about pronouns and their *antecedents* (those NP positions to which they co-refer) still hold in multi-clause constructions? It appears that it does, because in (70) the anaphor *himself* co-refers with an NP (*Scott*) within its own clause, and seems well-formed. However, the anaphor in (71) co-refers with the subject of the matrix clause (*Rico*) and seems ungrammatical (*himself* does not refer to *Rico*). Thus an anaphor (i.e. reflexive pronoun) requires reference within its local clause. In (72) the pronominal element *him* co-refers with the subject of the matrix clause (*Rico*) and seems well-formed, yet in (73) *him* co-refers (or is co-indexed) with the subject of the embedded clause (*Scott*) and indeed seems ungrammatical. Thus, pronominals seem not to require reference within a local clause. It also turns out that the personal pronoun does not have to co-refer with the subject of the matrix clause, as it does in (72). If we 'strip' off the co-index from the subject NP (*Rico*), the interpretation of the construction would be that the personal pronoun *him* would refer to someone other than *Rico*, someone mentioned in the discourse, perhaps. Importantly, the generalization about personal pronouns still holds, however, because the pronoun would not get its reference in its own clause. Finally, (74) shows that the referential expression (R-expression) *Lola* does not co-refer with any other position, and thus cannot be co-indexed with any position in the sentence.

Given these data and the notions of c-command and Government described in the section on *Structural Relations*, the following describes more formally the principles of the Binding Theory:

75. Binding Theory:

X binds Y if and only if X c-commands Y and X and Y are co-indexed.

Principle A: An anaphor must be bound in its governing category (it must be c-commanded by an antecedent with which it is co-indexed)
Principle B: A pronominal must be free in its governing category (it must not be c-commanded within the same clause)
Principle C: An R-expression (lexical NP) must be free everywhere (it must not be c-commanded by anything)

A *governing category* is the smallest domain (NP or CP) that contains the anaphor/pronominal and its governor (see (30) for a definition of Government). In (70) the anaphor *himself is* c-commanded by the subject of the embedded clause (*Scott*) and co-indexed with it. Therefore, it is bound in its governing category, which is the bracketed CP. Yet in (71) the anaphor is not c-commanded by the subject of the matrix clause (*Rico*). Because an anaphor must be bound in its governing category, (71) is ruled out by Principle A of the Binding Theory. In (72) the pronominal element *him* is not c-commanded by its antecedent *Rico*, and thus is free in its governing category. Yet in (73) the pronoun is bound in its governing category, but because it is a pronoun (which must be free in its governing category) and not a reflexive, (73) is ruled out by Principle B. Finally, in (74) the R-expression *Lola* is not c-commanded and co-indexed with any position.

The ECP and its relation to Binding

The ECP (63) also suggests that there are similarities between the theories of Binding and Traces, because both theories refer to the notion of Government. Indeed, it turns out that what holds for overt NPs also holds for 'empty' NPs or traces. We should expect this because both empty and phonologically realized categories are similar distributionally (i.e. they occur in the same positions) and share similar properties. Therefore, the principles of Binding also appear to hold for traces. Starting with Principle A (75), an anaphor (e.g. *herself*) must be bound in its governing category (roughly, within its own clause); so too must an NP-trace be bound in its governing category. Principle B states that a pronominal (e.g. *her*) must be free in its governing category. Although there are no empty categories in English that have this property, there is an empty category *pro* (or 'little pro') that indeed does so in other languages (e.g. Spanish, Italian). These languages allow the pronoun to be 'dropped' (hence the term *pro-drop languages*), yielding an empty category having all the properties of the lexically filled pronoun. Finally, Principle C states that an R-expression (e.g. *Lola*) must be free everywhere; so too must a *wh*-trace be free.

Features and their role in Binding

We have been assuming that lexical and functional categories are *primitives*; that is, they cannot be further decomposed. However, the theory suggests otherwise, and that, indeed, categories can be decomposed into a set of *features* and that these features specify what the categories have in common. For example, the lexical categories noun (N), verb (V), adjective (A), and preposition (P) can each be described in terms of a unique *feature complex*:

76. $N = [+N, -V]$
    $V = [N, +V]$
    $A = [+N, +V]$
    $P = [-N, -V]$

Note that the categories V and P each are designated by the [–N] feature. This suggests that they behave similarly, and, indeed, they both assign Case and Theta-roles to their complements. Similarly, INFL can have the feature [±TNS]. INFL marked as [+TNS] assigns Case to its subject; INFL marked as [–TNS] does not. C (Comp) is also considered by some to be assigned the feature [±Wh], thus either heading an embedded interrogative [+Wh] or an embedded clause [–Wh].

The Binding principles just described also interact with feature complexes. Reflexive pronouns, subject to Principle A, are said to have the feature complex [+Anaphor, –Pronominal]. Personal pronouns, subject to Principle B, have the feature complex [–Anaphor, +Pronominal]. Referential expressions, subject to Principle C, have the features [–Anaphor, –Pronominal]. Thus, the Binding Theory has often been recast into the following:

• An element that has the feature [+Anaphor] must be bound in its governing category.
• An element that has the feature [+Pronominal] must be free in its governing category.
• An element that has the features [–Anaphor, –Pronominal] must be free.

Finally, non-overt categories (e.g. *wh*-trace and NP-trace) can also be decomposed into sets of features. The idea here is that if features of Binding can characterize *overt* NPs, then they should also characterize *non-overt* NPs. Without delving into the details, recall that NP-movement (61) has an argument position landing site and yields an NP-trace. It turns out that the NP-trace is bound in its governing category, much like a reflexive pronoun with the feature [+Anaphor] is. Thus, both an anaphor and an NP-trace are subject to Principle A. *Wh*-movement has an A-bar (non-argument) position landing site and yields a *wh*-trace. Like an NP-trace, a *wh*-trace is c-commanded by its antecedent and is co-indexed with it; thus, it is also bound in its governing category. However, the Binding Theory is only concerned with binding from an A-position, and because the antecedent to the trace is in an A-bar position (Spec), it is *not A-bound* by anything in its governing category, just like an R-expression. Both an R-expression and a *wh*-trace, then, are subject to Principle C.

Principles and parameters

Some of the principles of the theory of syntax under consideration here are suggested to be part of Universal Grammar (UG), the part of the grammar that is innately given by virtue of our human genetic code and which constrains language acquisition. For example, the Head Principle, the Projection Principle, the Empty Category Principle, aspects of the Binding, X-bar and Trace Theories, the notions of d- and s-structure, are all assumed to be part of UG. Of course, languages are different, so it can't be that all languages treat these principles in exactly the same way. The aspect of the theory that captures the variation among languages is the notion of *parameters*. For example, the Head Principle states that each phrase must have a head that shares the same properties of the phrasal node projections. But it doesn't say anything about the *order* of the head to its complements. Evidence from English suggests that the head appears to the left of its complements or arguments, hence, English is a *head-initial* language. However, there are many languages where the head appears after its complements; these languages are known as *head-final* (e.g. Japanese). So, there is a two-choice parameter that the child is assumed to set given appropriate linguistic *triggers* (input). The same choice is made for the position of the Specifier and Adjunct Phrases. There are several other proposed parameters, including whether or not *wh*-movement is allowed by the grammar, whether or not pronouns can be omitted (the *pro-drop parameter*), the structural barriers to movement, and other features.[7]

Summary and implications for normal and disordered language

In this review of syntax, it was claimed that a native speaker's knowledge of language involves lexical and functional category representations, phrasal representations that can be ordered hierarchically to describe sentence structure (captured by the X-bar schema), the principles of c-command and Government that describe relations among nodes in the tree, the lexicon and properties of lexical items (Theta Theory and Case Theory) and how they contribute to, and interact with, syntax, d- and s-structure realizations of sentences along with transformations or movement rules that relate the two, the three principles of Binding Theory and how they related to Trace Theory, and feature complexes. Many of these theoretical constructs have had a profound impact on accounts of language acquisition, sentence production and sentence comprehension in both normal and disordered language users. A full discussion of this research is beyond the scope of the present chapter; however, the following examples taken from the literature are offered.

The Garden Path Theory of Sentence Processing (e.g. Frazier, 1978; Frazier and Clifton, 1995)

For almost two decades this work has shown how linguistic theory is unavoidably linked to accounts of human sentence processing. In brief, this account claims that the human sentence processor constructs tree structures using syntactic representations from X-bar Theory. The construction of these syntactic representations is constrained by various processing principles (e.g. *minimal attachment*: do not postulate any unnecessary nodes; *late closure*: attach new items into the clause or phrase currently being processed). This account is closely associated with the theory of *modularity*, whereby the language-processing system is claimed to consist of a number of independent, autonomous processors that do not interact until each has run its course of operation.

The Constraint Satisfaction Account of Sentence Processing (e.g. MacDonald, Pearlmutter and Seidenberg, 1994)

This work has also shown the inescapable link between linguistic theory and sentence processing. However, instead of focusing on syntactic representations, this account claims that lexical representations (e.g. thematic roles, semantic properties) are the primary source of establishing the structure and meaning of a sentence. Unlike the garden path account, this account is highly interactive because all information (e.g. semantic, pragmatic etc.) interacts initially during sentence processing.

Gap-filling

This is psycholinguistic terminology for the trace–antecedent relation. Swinney and colleagues (e.g. Swinney, Ford, Frauenfelder and Bresnan, 1989; Swinney and Osterhout, 1991) have found that when a lexically unfilled position (i.e. a trace) is encountered during the process of attempting to understand a sentence, that position is filled automatically and immediately by the legal antecedent, that is, by the co-indexed NP to which the unfilled position co-refers. Relatedly, Nicol (1988) has found that at the point where a reflexive pronoun is encountered in a sentence, only the grammatically appropriate, locally bound antecedent is accessed, and when a personal pronoun is encountered, only the non-locally bound antecedent is accessed.

Lexical representations

Shapiro and colleagues (Shapiro, Zurif and Grimshaw, 1987,1989; Shapiro, Brookins, Gordon and Nagel, 1991; see also Rubin, Newhoff, Peach and Shapiro, 1996) have found that when a verb is encountered in a sentence, all of the verb's argument structure possibilities are activated. Once argument structure information is made available to the system, most sentence processing accounts hypothesize an operation that then links thematic roles to arguments in the sentence.

Sentence comprehension in aphasia

Here there is a host of findings that are intimately tied to linguistic theory. One of the most important set of works that has shown the importance of linguistic theory to the description and explanation of aphasia is from Grodzinsky (1990, 1995b). Briefly, he has shown that the sentence comprehension patterns evinced by agrammatic Broca's aphasic patients can be described in terms of the deletion of traces (see also Hickok, Zurif and Canseco-Gonzales, 1993; Mauner, Fromkin and Cornell, 1993). Relatedly, Zurif and colleagues (Zurif, Swinney, Prather, Solomon and Bushell, 1993; Swinney and Zurif, 1995) have shown that their agrammatic Broca's aphasic patients do not normally reaccess the antecedent to a trace during sentence comprehension, yet their Wernicke's aphasic patients do. On the other hand, Shapiro, Gordon, Hack and Killackey (1993) have found that Wernicke's aphasic patients do not normally access the argument structure possibilities for verbs, yet Broca's aphasic patients do. This 'double-dissociation' suggests that the process of connecting a trace to its antecedent is independent from the process of accessing the argument-taking properties of the verb, and that, perhaps, different brain regions are responsible for the normal operation of each.

Sentence production in aphasia

Friedmann and Grodzinsky (1997), and Hagiwara (1995) have recently shown how the sentence production patterns of agrammatic aphasic patients can be described in terms of the phrase structure tree. For example, adopting the Split-Infl hypothesis, Friedmann and Grodzinsky propose that the different levels of severity observed in agrammatic production might be explained by where in the phrase-structure tree a defective node (e.g. Tense, Agreement, COMP) occurs; the lower the node in the tree, the more severe the impairment because the tree cannot project higher than the impaired node.

Treatment of language deficits

Thompson and colleagues (Thompson and Shapiro, 1994, 1995; Thompson, Shapiro, Ballard, Jacobs, Schneider and Tait, 1997) have shown in a series of studies that the lexical and syntactic properties of sentences need to be considered in treatment programs for agrammatic aphasia. Training production of complex structures that contain traces (e.g. *wh*-questions, relative clauses, passives) results not only in learning of trained structures, but also results in generalization to untrained sentences that share linguistic properties. For example, training *wh*-movement structures [e.g. *wh*-questions; see (60) above] generalizes to other structures relying on *wh*-movement (e.g. relative clauses) but not to structures relying on NP-movement [e.g. passives; see (59) above].

Language acquisition and language disorders in children

Several recent accounts of normal language acquisition have referred to X-bar Theory to explain the relatively impoverished use of functional categories in early grammar. For example, Lebeaux (1988) and Radford (1988) have claimed that early grammar lacks the functional projections DET, INFL and COMP. Thus, the difference between early and adult grammars is structural. Hyams (1996), however, has claimed that early grammar has intact functional projections, but that the projections are underspecified in terms of their link to the discourse. Relatedly, there have been several attempts to describe specific language impairment (SLI) in children by referring to the development of use of functional projections (e.g. Leonard, 1995; Rice, Wexler and Cleave, 1995).

There are, of course, many more examples of work that relate linguistic theory to language performance, far too numerous to do justice to here. The reader is referred to the recent special issues on Agrammatism in *Brain and Language* (1995) and to the *Journal of Psycholinguistic Research* (specifically, the special issues from the CUNY Human Sentence Processing Conference), *Language Acquisition*, as well as to articles in the *Journal of Speech and Hearing Research*.

To conclude, understanding much of the research in language acquisition, comprehension and production is difficult without at least an introductory knowledge of syntax. I hope that this introduction will serve as an entry into this research.

Acknowledgements

I would like to acknowledge the support from NIH (NIDCD) grants DC00494 and DC01948. 1 would also like to thank Dr Cynthia Thompson and two anonymous reviewers for their very helpful comments on an earlier draft of the paper from which this chapter originates.

Notes

1. There are several other influential linguistic theories, for example, Generalized Phrase Structure Grammar (GPSG) and its variants (e.g. Gazdar, Klein, Pullum and Sag, 1985), Lexical Functional Grammar (LFG) (Kaplan and Bresnan, 1982), Relational

Grammar (e.g. Perlmutter and Rosen, 1982) and Constructional Grammar (Fillmore, 1988; Goldberg, 1995). The reader is directed to Sells (1985) for a summary of some of these theories.

2. If the head occurs to the left of its complements in English, then what about the structure of NPs (e.g. *the mechanic*)? The article *the* seems to modify the N (*mechanic*), yet the 'head' Noun appears to its right. One possibility that has been suggested by Abney (1987) and that is favoured by many linguists is to consider NPs as Determiner Phrases (DPs), where the category DET is now the head of the DP and therefore falls to the left of its complement: DP →; DET N.

3. More recent analyses (e.g. Pollock, 1989) suggest that the INFL projection can be divided into separated phrases for Tense (TNS) and Agreement (AGR), and AGR subdivided into AGR-S (subject) and AGR-O (object). Each of these has a functional category as head. This modification has become known as the 'Split-Infl Hypothesis'.

4. More recently, the subject NP is claimed to be base generated *internally*, just like the direct and indirect object positions. That is, the subject NP is generated under VP projection and 'raises' to sentence-initial position, leaving behind a *trace* of that movement (Sportiche, 1988).

5. Verbs with two internal arguments (e.g. *double-object* verbs) present interesting problems for the binary branching hypothesis discussed in the section on X-bar Theory. Consider:

(i)   Joanna sent the letter to Mitzi.
(ii) Joanna sent Mitzi the letter.

(i) and (ii) appear to be related because they contain similar arguments and thematic roles, though the arguments in each appear in different syntactic positions. How does the theory account for these facts? Not so easily, it turns out. Recall that a head and its arguments are said to be 'sisters' (that is, they are on the same phrasal level in the tree), and that the head is said to c-command its arguments. Skipping the details, if binary branching is retained, only one argument can be sister to the head V, the other argument is attached to a V-bar; that is higher in the tree. Thus, in (i) V c-commands its argument NP *the letter*, but it doesn't c-command the second internal argument, the NP *Mitzi* in the PP *to Mitzi*. Relatedly, in (ii) a different argument is sister to the head (the NP *Mitzi*) whereas the second internal argument (*the letter*) attaches higher up in the tree and is not c-commanded by V. If both (i) and (ii) are related, as they indeed seem to be, then why should the head c-command a different argument in each case?

Various solutions have been proposed to account for double-object verbs. A full discussion of these issues is far beyond the scope of this chapter. The reader is referred to Barrs and Lasnik (1986), who suggest a 'flat' rather than a binary branching structure, and to Larson (1988) and Jackendoff (1990b) where the relations among various principles of the grammar and double-object verbs are explored.

6. There are two other levels of representation that will not be discussed in this chapter. One is Phonetic Form (PF), which is the stuff of Phonology and is part of the A–P (articulatory–phonetic) interface. The other is Logical Form (LF), which is concerned with semantic interpretation and scope of quantifiers and *wh*-phrases and is part of the C–I (conceptual–intentional) interface. Most of what holds at d- and s-structure also holds for LF, such as the Projection Principle and the Empty Category Principle.

7. Recently, Chomsky and colleagues have explored an account known as the Minimalist Program. The concern is with *economy of representation*. A basic assumption is that the theory should prefer complex structures to complex principles (from Larson, 1988). Practically, this means that trees are often far more complex than have

been characterized in this chapter (particularly because of a variant of Pollock's Split-Infl hypothesis) and, thus, some principles are no longer necessary. Briefly, s- and d-structure are eliminated, and so too are the principles that refer only to those levels of representation. For example, the Projection Principle and the Theta Criterion are no longer necessary because their existence is dependent on d-structure. And, because conditions that apply at s-structure also apply at LF, s-structure can be eliminated (LF is retained for independent reasons, specifically because it is at the conceptual–intentional interface). The Minimalist Program is considered preliminary and will surely undergo many changes. For details, the reader is referred to Chomsky (1995), a complex set of readings, and to Marantz (1995), a more accessible version.

Chapter 2
The processing of long-distance dependencies in normal listeners: Evidence for form-driven activation

LEWIS P. SHAPIRO

Introduction

In this chapter we discuss two recent studies that investigate on-line processing of long-distance dependencies using normal subjects. The investigation of how such structural processing operates under real-time constraints may be particularly illuminating for accounts of sentence processing. For example, we investigate how and when lexical properties (e.g. semantic entailments) influence the connection between two non-adjacent positions. Based on some support from the literature we initially assume that lexical properties do *not* influence *initial* structural processing; that is, we hypothesize that connecting non-adjacent positions during on-line sentence comprehension is a *form-driven* process – in this case, driven by the syntactic nature of the connection between the non-adjacent positions.

The first study that we describe investigates verb phrase (VP) -ellipsis constructions embedded with verbs that place severe constraints on their reference-taking properties. To forecast our case, we find that the semantic constraints that verb's place on final interpretation do not seem to influence on-line sentence analysis. The second study examines *who/what* versus *which*-noun phrase (NP) questions, the latter being *discourse-linked*. Here we find that on-line activation of the referents for pro-forms and empty categories occurs across discourse.

Study 1: Verb properties and gap-filling in complex VP-ellipsis constructions (Shapiro, Hestvik, Suzuki and Garcia, 1998)

Consider the following:
1. *The policeman*$_i$ defended himself$_i$, and *the fireman*$_j$ did ___$_{(?)}$ too, according to someone who was there.

35

This construction contains two clauses, *the policeman defended himself* and *the fireman did too*. The second clause contains a bare auxiliary – *did* – that indicates the elision of a VP; that elided VP gets its reference from the VP in the first clause. On some accounts (e.g. Lobeck, 1992; Shapiro and Hestvik, 1995) there is an empty category in the elided VP position that is subject to the same constraints any empty category is subject to, for example, Government and the Empty Category Principle (e.g. Chomsky, 1986a; see also Shapiro, 1997).

There are two interpretations of (1). The *sloppy* interpretation is that the 'fireman defended *himself*', where *himself* co-refers with *the fireman*; this interpretation is typically generated first by approximately 80% of normal listeners during an off-line judgment task and is set by the requirements of Principle A of Binding Theory (BT): an anaphor must be locally bound. The *strict* interpretation is that the 'fireman defended *him*', where *him* co-refers with *the policeman* – the subject of the initial clause; this interpretation is often more difficult to generate off-line (a majority of listeners do indeed make such an interpretation, though it is certainly not the first interpretation to come to mind; see Shapiro and Hestvik, 1995; Shapiro, Hestvik, Suzuki and Garcia, 1998) and is set by Principle B of BT: a pronoun must be free in its governing category.

In an on-line examination of such VP-ellipsis understanding, Shapiro and Hestvik (1995) found that normal listeners (re)activate the subject NP from the first, source clause (e.g. *the policeman*) at the elided VP position of the second clause (i.e. the gap). Because such an interpretation is obviously the less-frequent one that is available to listeners, we interpreted our results as reflecting the automatic, form-driven nature of gap-filling. In our most recent study that we describe here we extend our investigation of ellipsis by manipulating the properties of verbs. Specifically, we used verbs that *allow only the sloppy interpretation*. Consider:

2. The optometrist who had signed the release [1] form asserted herself [2], and the pilot who needed to pass [3] the training exam did [4] too ....

3. The gambler who won ten hands in [1] a row winked his [2] eyes, and the pit boss who was in on [3] the elaborate scheme did [4] too ....

In (2) the verb *assert* allows only the reflexive reading; that is, only the 'sloppy' interpretation is allowed in the second clause (the 'pilot' can only assert herself, and not the 'optometrist'). Similarly, in (2) the verb *wink* requires an object (a body part) that is possessed by the subject NP (the 'pit boss' cannot typically wink the 'gambler's' eyes). Though other continuations exist ('assert control', 'wink' as intransitive), we found that off-line judgments from an independent subject group presented with sentences like (2) and (3) revealed that only the sloppy interpretation was available. Thus, the lexical properties of these 'reflexive' and 'inalienable body-part possession' verbs (see, for example, Levin, 1994) place obvious constraints on the interpretation of VP-ellipsis constructions.

We investigated whether on-line gap-filling would respect these lexical constraints. This issue reflects on the basic nature of sentence processing. For example, in the constraint–satisfaction framework, probabilistic information (e.g. frequency-of-use), context and lexical properties work together to constrain interpretation (e.g. MacDonald, Pearlmutter and Seidenberg, 1994). Such an account would predict that only the sloppy reading would be active on-line, because it is (a) substantially more frequent overall in ellipsis constructions and (b) the lexical properties of the verb only allow the sloppy interpretation. However, a strongly form-driven account of gap-filling would predict that gap-filling is a reflexive, automatic process that initially ignores probabilistic and lexical constraints; such constraints are said to exert their influence after-the-fact (see, for example, Love and Swinney, 1996 and Shapiro, Swinney and Borsky, 1998). On this latter account, then, both the sloppy and strict interpretations should be available in the immediate temporal vicinity of the gap. And, it should only be after-the-fact that the context-appropriate interpretation is available.

We used the cross-modal priming (CMP) task. Sentences were presented to listeners over headphones. During the temporal unfolding of each sentence, a visual lexical decision probe (WORD/NONWORD) was presented for 500 ms at a strategically located probe position (in the test sentences). When the probe formed a word, it was related to either the subject from the first clause (strict interpretation), the subject from the second clause (sloppy interpretation), or was an unrelated control probe, matched to its related counterpart in terms of number of letters/syllables, frequency of occurrence, and base reaction times (RTs) (gathered from an independent group of subjects during a standard visual lexical decision task). When RTs to the related probes are significantly faster than RTs to the control probes, priming is said to have occurred, which suggests that a meaning related to the probe has been activated.

Predictions

Reflexive or inalienable possession verbs that only allow the sloppy interpretation off-line were inserted into VP-ellipsis constructions. We repeat here sentence (2):

The optometrist who had signed the release [1] form asserted herself [2], and the pilot who needed to pass [3] the training exam did [4] too
....

In one experiment we examined whether listeners would reactivate the subject NP from the *first* clause (e.g. *the optometrist*); this pattern would indicate that listeners generate the strict reading on-line. Additionally in this experiment we examined whether listeners access the locally bound antecedent for the reflexive. In this case, we should observe significant priming for *the optometrist* at the reflexive ([2]), yet find no priming at the pre-reflexive position ([1]). In a second experiment we considered whether listeners would reactivate the subject NP from the *second* clause in the test sentences (i.e. the sloppy interpretation). Thus, if we observe priming for, for example, *the pilot* at the elided VP position ([4]), yet observe no priming at the pre-gap position ([3]), then the subject NP from the second clause will have been *re*accessed at the gap.

Subjects included 96 college-age neurologically intact adults; 16 each were randomly assigned to each probe position for each experiment (strict interpretation, sloppy interpretation). Each subject received both a control and related probe for each sentence (nested, and presented two weeks apart). All probes (word and non-word) except those associated with the test sentences were randomly distributed across different temporal positions in the sentences. For the test sentences of Experiment 1 (strict interpretation), there were four probe positions; for Experiment 2 (sloppy interpretation) there were two probe positions. The sentences were presented over headphones through a DAT player. During the course of each sentence, a lexical decision probe appeared momentarily on the screen. Subjects were required to attend to the sentences and make a lexical decision quickly and accurately by pressing one of two response keys (WORD, NONWORD); RTs to this decision were recorded by the computer. In approximately 20% of the trials, the tape was stopped and subjects were asked to paraphrase the sentence that they had just heard. RTLab software controlled stimulus presentation and timing.

Results of, and discussion on, Study 1

Only correct responses to the real word probes presented with test sentences were used in the analyses. RTs greater than 2000 ms were discarded as errors. We first present the data from Experiment 1 (strict interpretation), shown in Table 2.1.

These data show the following patterns: at position 1 – the pre-reflexive probe point – no significant priming was observed; that is, RTs to the related probes (related to the subject NP from the first clause) were not significantly faster than to their controls. However, at position 2 – the reflexive – significant priming was observed. Thus, when a reflexive is encountered in a sentence, the locally bound NP to which it co-refers is reactivated (see also Nicol, 1988). More to the purposes of the experiment, at position 3 – the pre-gap position in the second clause – significant priming was not observed. However, at position 4 – the gap or elided VP position – significantly faster RTs to the related probes (related, again, to the subject NP from the first clause, i.e. the strict interpretation) was observed relative to the RTs for the control probes.

Table 2.1. Results of Experiment 1 (strict interpretation)

	Results (in ms): Strict	
Positions	Control	Related
1 (pre-reflexive)	722	712
2 (reflexive)	755	721*
3 (pre-gap)	719	710
4 (gap)	801	769*

*$p < 0.01$.

The results from Experiment 2 are shown in Table 2.2.

Table 2.2. Results of Experiment 2 (sloppy interpretation)

	Results (in ms): Sloppy	
Positions	Control	Related
3 (pre-gap)	808	801
4 (gap)	855	829*

*$p < 0.01$.

The data from this experiment show that at position 3 – the pre-gap position – no significant priming was observed. That is, the RTs for the control probes and for the related probes (related to the subject NP from the second clause; i.e. the sloppy interpretation) were not significantly different. However, at probe position 4 – the gap or elided VP – RTs to probes related to the subject NP were, again, significantly faster than RTs to controls.

Putting the data from both experiments together, listeners apparently reaccess the subject NP from both the first and second clauses at the elided VP position in the second clause. Thus, they have available *both* the sloppy and strict interpretation on-line (see Hickok, 1993 and Nicol and Pickering, 1993, for further evidence suggesting multiple access of *structural* possibilities). The implications for accounts of sentence processing are clear. Given that (1) the verbs inserted into these constructions were highly constrained towards only the sloppy interpretation, and that (2) off-line judgments suggest that only the sloppy interpretation is available to listeners (note that even with verbs that allow both interpretations, the sloppy reading is chosen initially by a wide majority of listeners; Shapiro and Hestvik, 1995), immediate structural processing appears to initially ignore such constraints. Yet, because listeners indeed generate solely the sloppy interpretation off-line, at a point between the gap and final interpretation listeners discard (or suppress) the strict reading. We suggest, therefore, that theories of sentence processing will have to include operations geared to (1) initial form-driven activation and (2) multiple interpretations. An account that claims multiple constraints initially converge on a single interpretation will need to be revised.

Study 2: *Who-what* and *which*-NP Questions
(Shapiro, Oster, Garcia, Massey and Thompson, 1999)

We now describe two experiments that extend the investigation of long-distance dependencies by examining the on-line processing of two different types of *wh*-questions: questions headed by *who* or *what* (e.g. *Who* did the policeman push___ into the street?) and questions headed by *which*-NP (e.g. *which student* did the policeman push ___ into the street?). These two types of *wh*-questions can be distinguished on linguistic grounds. For example, *which* phrases are considered *referential* (i.e. they include participants taking part in the event described, e.g. *student*) whereas *who* and *what* questions are considered *non-referential*. Perhaps related to their referentiality, *which* phrases pick out an individual from a set of individuals explicitly mentioned or inferred from the discourse and are therefore considered *discourse-linked* (*D-linked*), whereas *who* and *what* phrases do not have to be.

We summarize these differences and examine their implications for sentence processing. De Vincenzi (1996) and Hickok and Avrutin (1995) have recently shown that these two question types are, indeed, differentiated in off-line sentence interpretation. Unlike their efforts, however, we focus on the processes that occur *prior* to final interpretation; we investigate on-line performance. In doing so, we interpret our data in terms of a sentence processing account that integrates discourse representations in putatively automatic operations of the parser.

A brief linguistic background

Consider the following:

4. Who-1 did Dillon push e-1?

According to Government-Binding, the *wh*-word *who* originates in the post-verb direct-object position and moves to a pre-verb position via the *transformation Move-alpha*. An empty category ('e') – a *trace* – is inserted into the post-verb position. The trace and moved category form a *dependency* relation (note that we are using numerals attached to positions to indicate that the positions relate to each other). The syntactic structure that exists before the NP is moved is known as the *d-structure* and that which exists after the NP is moved is the *s-structure*. Consider, then, the derivation (from d- to s-structure) of the *wh*-question in (4) (see Figure 2.1).

5.

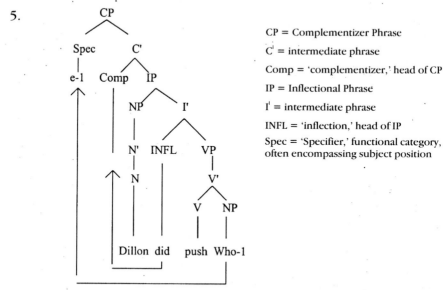

CP = Complementizer Phrase

C' = intermediate phrase

Comp = 'complementizer,' head of CP

IP = Inflectional Phrase

I' = intermediate phrase

INFL = 'inflection,' head of IP

Spec = 'Specifier,' functional category, often encompassing subject position

Figure 2.1

Skipping some details, when *who* moves out of its direct-object position (the NP immediately dominated by V'), it will leave behind a trace; the trace and the moved NP, *who* – which has moved to Spec of CP – form a *trace-antecedent dependency* or *chain*. Furthermore, there is another movement in (5), where INFL (*did*) 'raises' to Comp. This *head-to-head* movement is mostly irrelevant for present purposes, but note that when two dependencies occur in one structure, one must be nested within the other for the sentence to be well formed (in this case, the dependency formed when *did* moves to Comp is nested within the dependency formed when *who* moves to Spec). Note also that Comp and Spec are non-argument positions (*A-bar* positions); these positions do not receive thematic roles directly; argument positions (*A* positions) – those that do receive thematic roles (like Agent and Patient, for example) – are, typically, subject and object NPs and objects of prepositions.

Finally, a constraint on the distribution of traces and antecedents requires that antecedents *c-command* their traces. A node X c-commands a node Y if and only if the first branching node dominating X also dominates Y. Using (5) as an example, we see that Spec of CP (to where *who* has moved) c-commands its trace, the direct-object NP position (immediately dominated by the V'), because the first branching node dominating Spec – CP – also dominates the NP. Note that the Comp position where the auxiliary *did* moved also c-commands its trace at INFL.

There is another level of representation – *Logical Form* (LF) – that enters into our discussion. LF is considered part of the conceptual–intentional interface; it is concerned with semantic interpretation and scope of quantifiers and *wh* phrases. Movement of *wh* phrases also occurs at LF (this movement is sometimes known as *Quantifier raising*). Consider the following:

6. Dillon pushed Joelle
7. Who did Dillon push?

The argument *Dillon* in (6) has an exact interpretation; it has one and only one referent (*Dillon*). However, the *wh* phrase *Who* in (7) has a *variable* interpretation; it does not, in principle, have a specific referent. Borrowing from standard logic, *who* is said to be an *operator* that binds a variable, x, as in:

8. *Who*$_i$ did Dillon push x_i

(8) is an LF representation (note that in LF, the trace is signified by a variable, x). In standard logic the operator takes *scope* over its domain; that is, operators can affect the interpretation of other elements. In this case, the *wh*-word – the operator – determines the interpretation of the entire sentence (that is, the sentence is an interrogative just because the operator is a *wh*-word). The scope domain of the operator is the domain which it c-commands [the CP, or clause; see (5)]. Hence, positions occupied by operators are left-peripheral because they must take scope over their domain. This means that every operator will need to move out of an argument position to a scope position. Basically, for *wh*-questions in English, this forces leftward movement of the operator (e.g. *who*) to an A-bar position [e.g. Spec of CP; see (5)].

The distinction between *who/what* and *which*-NP questions

With this background in mind, in this section we briefly review linguistic evidence that supports a distinction between *who/what* questions and *which*-NP questions.

D-linking

We begin with Pesetsky's (1987) observation that *which*-phrases, unlike *who* or *what*, are *D-linked*. Consider:

9. Which woman did the soldier push into the street?
10. Who did the soldier push into the street?

The question in (9) presupposes a *set* of women, one of whom was pushed into the street. In (10) no such presupposition is required for interpretation. Thus, (9) would be infelicitous without a discourse (overt, or covert) to pick an individual out from a set of individuals; in (10) no set of individuals need be presumed. This distinction is made clear when you attempt to add a phrase like *the hell* (as in, *Who [the hell] did the soldier push into the street?*), which expresses ignorance of the possible answers to (10), suggesting an isolation from any possible discourse. Note that adding such a phrase is incompatible with the discourse-linked representation set up with (9) (*Which woman [the hell] did the soldier push into the street?*).

Furthermore, Pesetsky claims that *D-linked wh-phrases are not operators*. Recall that every operator must occupy an A-bar position at LF because it must have scope over its domain, thereby requiring movement. If *which*-NPs are not operators, they do not have to move at LF. The claim that D-linked *which*-NPs are not operators makes a great deal of sense given that operators bind variables that have *non-referential* interpretations. NPs that pick out a referent from the universe of discourse [*Dillon*, in (6), for example] do not enter into the operator-variable dependency, and neither should *which*-NPs that also pick out a referent from the discourse. Thus, whether or not a phrase is D-linked is concomitant with whether or not the phrase is considered referential.

Binding and Government

Rizzi (1990) uses the notion of referentiality to explain the distinction between traces and antecedents that connect via *Binding* and those that connect via *Government*. In essence, only the dependency between phrases and antecedents that bear a referential *index* enter into Binding, whereas those not bearing such an index connect via *Government*. Again, if an argument refers to participants in the event, then that argument is said to be referential. If that argument moves, it forms a dependency with its trace. The antecedent (moved NP) *binds* the trace if it c-commands the trace, and if both the antecedent and the trace are *co-indexed*. However, on Rizzi's account a moved argument that is not referential – that does not refer to a participant in the event – cannot be identified by Binding because it cannot bear a referential index. Instead, the antecedent is said to *govern* its trace. *Government* is a local relation among nodes in a tree. The antecedent governs the trace if it c-commands it, and if no other potential governor intervenes between the two positions (typically, a governor is a head). This distinction allows for a long-distance relation between a trace and its antecedent in the case of a binding relation. The Government relation is more local, and sometimes requires 'short' moves (because the antecedent cannot cross an intervening potential governor, or *barrier*) that leave multiple traces along the path travelled by the moved NP.

Most importantly, Cinque (1990) extends Rizzi's framework explicitly to describe the differences between *which*-NPs and *who* and *what* phrases. Again, *which*-NP phrases are intrinsically referential – are D-linked; they therefore enter into binding dependencies. *Who* and *what* phrases are non-referential – are not D-linked; they enter into Government chains. Thus, long-distance movement is allowed with *which*-NPs and only short, cyclical movement is allowed with *who* and *what* phrases.

Linguistic distinctions and their relevance to processing

What are we to make of the linguistic work that suggests various ways to cut the pie regarding *which*-NPs and *who* and *what* phrases? To review, *which*-phrases are referential and therefore do not enter into operator-variable dependencies at LF; *who* and *what* questions are potentially not referential and therefore are operators that do bind variables. *Which*-NPs are D-linked; *who* and *what* questions are potentially not. *Which*-NPs result in dependencies that are explained via Binding; *who* and *what* form Government chains.

Our concern here is, of course, with language processing. Given, however, that there are several linguistic facets to the distinction between *which*-NPs and *who* and *what* questions, we might ask which – if any – could be relevant to any predicted distinction in terms of on-line processing. Our intuitions – buttressed by some psycholinguistic evidence (see below) – suggest that the relevant notion that distinguishes these two types of *wh*-questions has to do with the D-linking properties of *which*-NP phrases and their referential quality. That is, it is the fact that *which*-NPs refer to selected individuals picked out from a set of individuals set up in the discourse – whereas *who* and *what* NPs do not have this property – that may have important implications for processing.

Let us be a bit more clear here about the distinction: *which*-NP questions are referential and carry an existential presupposition that requires a connection to the discourse. Based on the linguistic literature we have been claiming that *who* and *what* questions are not referential and are not D-linked. Yet, on simple reflection *who* and *what* questions can, indeed, refer to a set of individuals constructed on the basis of the discourse, just like *which*-NP questions. For example, if we ask a particular group of people 'who wants ice cream?' we likely don't mean something like 'who in the world wants ice cream?' Instead, we mean: 'of this group of people stipulated in the world of discourse, who among this group wants ice cream?' However, our review suggests that the grammar *requires* that *which*-NP questions be D-linked (indeed, *which*-NP questions are infelicitous without a discourse), whereas *who* and *what* questions *may or may not be*.

To forecast our case, then, we assume that if the grammar *requires* a link to the discourse, this will add a burden to the sentence processor (see also Shapiro and Hestvik, 1995); that burden will be reflected in a particular pattern of results that differentiates *which*-NP constructions from their *who* and *what* counterparts on-line.

We now report on two experiments. The first involves *who* and *what* questions, the second, *which*-NP questions. The initial hypothesis is that the sentence-processing system will respect the grammar in the following way. Based on past gap-filling work, we predict that immediate gap-filling effects will be observed with *who* and *what* questions. However, with *which*-NP constructions, we will observe a different, delayed, time-course of gap-filling. This prediction is based on the structural differences between the two types of dependencies outlined in the introduction, and, in particular, the D-linking and referential nature that is required of *which*-NP constructions.

Experiment 1: *Who* and *What* questions

Consider the following example from our first experiment:

11. The soldier is pushing *the unruly student* violently into the street?
    Who [1] is the soldier [2] pushing ___ [3] violently [4] into the street?

Note that there is a gap in the direct-object position occurring after the verb 'pushing'. The gap gets its reference from the *wh*-word 'who', which, in turn, depends on the explicitly mentioned direct object from the first sentence, 'the unruly student'. Thus, to understand the discourse, a listener must connect the empty direct-object position after the verb in the question to the *wh*-word that comes before it, and must also connect the *wh*-word to the direct object from the initial sentence. To the best of our knowledge, there have been no published reports on how listeners process such constructions on-line. How listeners do this, of course, will have important implications for accounts of normal sentence processing. For example, the gap (position [3]) is a long distance from the explicit referent; indeed, the referent and gap are separated by a sentence boundary, and a few phrasal and clausal boundaries as well. One can imagine that the referent is simply too far away to be activated at the gap. However, note that there is a *wh*-word (a pro-form) at the beginning of the question that in fact gets its reference from the direct object in the first sentence. And by various syntactic accounts, we know that the *wh*-word and the gap also co-refer. Thus, in essence, there are three elements – the explicitly mentioned direct object in the first sentence, the *wh*-word and the gap (both in the second sentence) – that form a *chain*. The question is, will we observe activation of the referent through the links of that chain?

We used the CMP task. Listeners were presented with spoken sentences like (11). The listener – while attending to the sentences – had to decide rapidly and accurately whether a visually presented lexical decision probe formed a word or non-word. RTs to this lexical decision were recorded. The lexical decision probes were either (a) semantically related to the direct object of the initial sentence (in the example above the related probe was SCHOOL, related to the direct object, *student*), (b) an unrelated control probe – controlled for frequency of occurrence, number of letters/syllables, and base RTs, or (c) non-words that conformed to orthographic rules of English.

In this experiment there were four probe positions, one occurring at the *wh*-word, one before the *wh*-gap, one occurring at the gap, and one occurring downstream from the gap. Normal listeners (15 subjects each) were randomly assigned to one of each probe position. Again, when RTs to the related probe are significantly faster than the RTs to the unrelated, control probes, *priming* is said to have occurred, which is evidence that the sense of the target word (in this case, *student*) has been activated in the immediate temporal vicinity of the probe.

Specifically, then, in this experiment we predicted the following patterns: because *who* functions much like a pronoun, we predicted activation of the referent of that 'pro-form' at who [1] – e.g. the direct object from the preceding sentence. However, given that there is no apparent way for the processor to 'know' that *who* indeed refers to something mentioned in the previous sentence at the temporal point when *who* is encountered, it is possible that no priming would occur for probes related to the direct object. No significant differences between the related and control probe were predicted at the pre-gap position [2], yet significantly faster RTs to the related probe relative to the unrelated probe at the gap position [3]. Such a pattern would indicate *reaccess* of the gap's filler.

Results of, and discussion on, Experiment 1

Table 2.3. Mean RTs (and SDs), in ms, to cross-modal lexical decision, *Who-what*

	Probe position			
Probes	*wh*-Word	Pre-gap	Gap	Post-gap
Control	847 (134)	747 (106)	793 (87)	802 (109)
Related	764* (162)	758 (99)	734* (76)	769 (152)

* significant for both subjects and items, $p < 0.01$.

We found significantly faster RTs to probes related to the direct object from the carrier phrase (764 ms) than to control probes (847 ms), at the *wh*-word. No priming was observed at the pre-gap position. Significantly faster RTs to the related probe (734 ms) were again found relative to control probes (793 ms) at the gap position. Note also that RTs to the control probes presented at the pre-gap position (747 ms) were significantly faster than the RTs to control probes presented at the gap position (793 ms).

The data, then, show that at position [1] – the *wh*-word – activation for the direct object from the preceding sentence was observed, suggesting that the *wh*-word acts like a pronoun and reactivates its possible antecedents. There are two limitations to this interpretation, however. First, note that we did not have a pre-*wh*-word probe position, so we cannot be sure that the direct object simply continues to be activated *across* the sentence boundary, and we fortuitously captured this continuous activation by probing at the *wh*-word. Secondly, if the *wh*-word indeed functions like a pro-form, then we would also expect activation of *any* NP (for example, the subject NP from the first clause); we are currently assessing both possibilities in further experimentation.

More pertinent to the focus of this chapter, however, are the patterns observed at both the pre-gap and gap positions. At the pre-gap position significant differences between the related and control probes were not observed, suggesting that the probes were well-controlled for base RTs. At the gap position we observed significantly faster RTs to the related compared to the control probes, strongly suggesting that when a listener encounters a direct-object gap in a *wh*-question, that gap is filled immediately by the grammatically appropriate antecedent. Furthermore, such gap-filling occurs across sentential boundaries. That is, when the NP to which the *wh*-gap refers [e.g. *the student* in example (8)] is located in a sentence that occurs prior to the *wh*-question, that NP is *reaccessed*. This gap-filling effect also appears to result in a larger interference effect when considering RTs to the control probes only; RTs to the control probes were significantly longer when the probes were presented at the gap than when presented at the pre-gap position. We will reserve further interpretation of these data until after we present our next experiment.

Experiment 2: *Which*-NP questions

In this experiment we changed the question form to *which* NP; the NP referred to was in the direct-object position of the declarative sentence. For example:

12. The soldier is pushing *the unruly student* violently into the street?
    Which student [1] is the soldier [2] pushing ____[3] violently [4] into the street?

In this experiment there were again four probe positions: One at the *wh*-word, at a pre-gap position, gap position and post-gap position. Fourteen subjects each were randomly assigned to each position. The first prediction is straightforward: at the *wh*-word we should observe significantly faster RTs to probes related to the *which*-NP (and thus to the direct object from the first sentence) relative to control probes. Next, if, when encountering a gap in a *which*-NP question, the antecedent to the gap is immediately reaccessed, then significantly faster RTs to the related relative to the unrelated control probes should be observed at the gap, but not at the pre-gap, position. Such a result would suggest that though there is linguistic evidence that *who* and *what* questions are dissimilar to *which*-NP questions, the parser treats them as similar objects. Another possibility makes a more direct connection to the grammar. If *which*-NP questions are indeed unlike *who* and *what* questions, then the time-course of activation of the antecedent may be different in the two cases. Specifically, if we assume that D-linking is required to connect the gap with its antecedent, and the antecedent to the direct object mentioned in the discourse, then gap-filling will be delayed because of the increased use of processing resources (see also Avrutin, in press; Frazier and McNamara, 1995 and Kluender, 1998, for similar arguments involving increased load for 'referential' processing).

Results of, and discussion on, Experiment 2

Table 2.4. Mean RTs (and SDs), in ms, to cross-modal lexical decision, *Which*-NP

		Probe position		
Probes	*Which*-NP	Pre-gap	Gap	Post-gap
Control	798 (97)	772 (93)	795 (52)	820 (139)
Related	709 (92)**	779 (93)	772 (66)	758* (81)

* significant ($p < 0.01$) for both subjects and items.
** significant ($p < 0.05$) for both subjects and items.

First, we observed significantly faster RTs to the related (709 ms) as compared to the control probes (798 ms) at the *which*-NP probe position, signifying lexical activation. Next, at the pre-gap position, no priming was observed. At the gap position, RTs to the related probes (772 ms) were faster than RTs to the unrelated control probes (795 ms), though this difference was significant at the 0.06 level. Finally, at the post-gap position significantly faster RTs were observed for related (758 ms) compared to the control (820 ms) probes.

The data from Experiment 2, then, showed that at the gap position there was a 'near-significant' trend. Yet, at the post-gap position significant RT differences were observed. Thus, at the downstream post-gap position there was unambiguous evidence that listeners reaccessed the antecedent to the gap. These patterns, then, were somewhat unlike those found in Experiment 1, where significant priming was found, unambiguously, at the gap. We interpret these data as evidence for delayed gap-filling in certain constructions; in the present case listeners fill *which*-NP gaps later in the temporal unfolding of the sentence than they fill *who* and *what* gaps. The question, of course, is why? Our initial answer has to do with the fact that *which*-NP constructions are required to be referential and D-linked; *who* and *what* questions are not. We assume that making contact with a discourse level of representation takes time and effort – perhaps extending the time-course of reaccess of the antecedent.

Before we continue with this interpretation – and consider additional supporting evidence – we need to consider the following apparent caveat: both experiments used a carrier phrase that set up a discourse to which the *wh*-gap (*who*, *what* or *which*-NP) could refer (for example, 'The soldier is pushing *the unruly student* violently into the street? *Who/Which* student is the soldier pushing violently into the street?'). And, we found immediate reaccess in *who* and *what* questions of an NP that occurred in that discourse. Thus, it could be argued that in practice, both types of *wh*-questions are discourse-linked (as we stated earlier). However, we assume that it is the grammatical distinction of the *wh*-questions that is at issue here, and not solely whether a discourse is presented. That is, *which*-NP questions are *required* to be D-linked because of their referential nature. Though *who* and *what* questions *can* refer to an entity mentioned in the discourse, in principle they are non-referential and thus do not have to be discourse-bound. It is this unmarked case – that *which*-NP questions must be D-linked but *what* and *who* questions do not have to be – that the parser appears to respect.

Our interpretation is supported by evidence from studies of both normal and brain-damaged subjects. For example, in our recent set of experiments examining gap-filling in complex VP-ellipsis structures, Shapiro and Hestvik (1995) showed that in coordinated ellipsis ('The policeman defended himself, *and* the fireman did ___ too, according to someone who was there'), gap-filling was observed in the immediate vicinity of the elided VP (after *did*). However, in subordinated ellipsis ('The policeman defended himself *because* the fireman did ___, according to someone who was there'), delayed gap-filling was observed (after *someone*). We suggested that in the coordinated case, gap-filling is driven by the syntactic nature of the trace-antecedent relation. In the subordinated case, however, to interpret the second, target, clause locally, a causal relation must also be computed between the two clauses; that is, X happened just *because* Y happened. Computing this causal relation stems from either a semantic or discourse representation (see, for example, Dalrymple, 1991; Kehler, 1994).

In effect, then, we are suggesting that when gap-filling is driven solely by syntactic considerations, immediate effects are observed. But when extra-syntactic information is involved, gap-filling is delayed. Our interpretation is buttressed by the work of De Vincenzi (1996). In Italian *wh*-questions can be ambiguous between subject- and object-extraction. These structures can be disambiguated, perhaps, by plausibility, that is, whether or not a post-verb NP is a better subject or a better object. De Vincenzi found a processing distinction between *who* and *which*-NP questions using a self-paced reading task where the reading material was segmented. Relatedly, Hickok and Avrutin (1995) found that their agrammatic aphasic patients showed a subject-object asymmetry only for *which*-NP questions, and not for *who* questions. And Avrutin (1998), examining both children and aphasic patients, has recently suggested that the most 'energy-consuming' operations are those that involve the interface between the syntactic and discourse modules of the language faculty, just the sort of suggestion we are making here. And finally, Frazier and McNamara (1995), using a grammaticality judgment rating task, found some indication that *which* and *who* questions are treated differently by aphasic patients. Their patients accepted significantly less grammatical object-gap *which* questions than normal controls, yet showed no difference in this regard with grammatical object-gap *who* questions. Also, these patients showed an asymmetry between subject- and object-extraction for *which* questions, but not for *who* questions. They suggest a 'Favour Referential Principle' in agrammatic aphasia, whereby these patients have a resource capacity limitation. When encountering both the computational syntactic demands of a complex sentence and the referential demands imposed by the content of the sentence, the aphasic listener favours the referential over the syntactic. This means that because they have both the referential and syntactic demands of the *which*-NP constructions to deal with – and assuming that the syntactic representation normally degrades rapidly – they will do worse than with non-referential *who* questions – those that must be represented syntactically.

Acknowledgements

The research reported in this manuscript was supported by NIH grant DC00494.

Chapter 3
Neuroanatomical organization of sentential processing operations: Evidence from aphasia on the (modular) processing of discontinuous dependencies

DAVID SWINNEY, TRACY LOVE, JANET NICOL, VIKKI BOUCK
AND LEA ANN HALD

Introduction

Our current understanding of the neuroanatomical organization of human language processing has been derived nearly in its entirety from observation and studies of language disorder arising from brain damage – from studies of aphasia. However, due to the ever-evolving behavioural description of language itself, our evolving understanding of the attendant cognitive processing resources underlying language, and our increasingly detailed knowledge of brain architecture, a 'final' description of the neuroanatomical organization of language is far from within our grasp. This chapter attempts to move toward a more complete description of language representation in the brain by focusing on processing at the level of description where language structure, processing resources and brain architecture are all most apparent – the level of sentence comprehension. In this chapter, we examine a specific (and demonstrably modular) process in comprehension – the processing of discontinuous dependencies – in normal and aphasic adults, and we detail the nature and time-course of this processing system as revealed by patterns of mental activation in these populations. Ultimately, we link a failure in the processing of these dependency relationships in certain brain-damaged populations to a neurologically localizable and elemental processing disruption, therein providing a basis for inferring how different brain regions subserve aspects of language comprehension. We will first discuss the types of intra-sentential relationships that will be the focus of this chapter, followed by a consideration of methodological issues that are central in any attempt to examine 'natural' language processing. Then we will present processing evidence from non-brain-damaged populations in dealing with these sentence-level relationships, and conclude with presentation of evidence from aphasia about the processing (or lack of processing) of these same relationships.

Background issues: the nature of dependency relationships

Language is rife with a variety of types of dependency relationships which are generally termed 'discontinuous' or 'long-distance'. We will deal with two classes of these in this chapter. The first, co-referential relationships, are concerned with relationships such as that which holds between a pronoun and its antecedent, as in the sentence:

1. The baker told the waitress at the restaurant that he would be late for work.

Here, the pronoun 'he' refers to the antecedent 'baker'. The question for the processor, of course, is how and when during processing the link between two dependent elements which are some distance apart (here, 'he' and 'baker') is accomplished.

The second type of long-distance dependency relationship which will concern us is structurally based – i.e. based on the fact that elements which are believed to be directly linked (and represented contiguously) in the 'underlying' or canonical representation of a language can be separated in surface forms of the language. For example, consider the object-relative construction in English:

2. The baker talked to the waitress who the customer accused of rude behaviour.

Two underlying sentences (propositions) comprise this complex sentence:

2a. The baker talked to the waitress.
2b. The customer accused the waitress of rude behaviour.

Note that in each 'underlying' sentence there is a canonical Subject–Verb–Object word order (this holds particularly for English, which is a strong S–V–O word-order language, and is more debatable for languages that allow various orderings of subjects, verbs and objects in declarative sentences). Thus, in the surface form of this complex sentence, the object (*waitress*) of the verb (*accused*) actually occurs *in front of* that verb (along with the relative pronoun 'who'); the verb and object are non-contiguous and out of order with regard to the underlying or 'canonical' order of basic relationships in the sentence. Various theoretical approaches to describing the relationships in such sentences have held that the surface order of the complex sentence is a result of 'movement' of the direct object from its canonical position.[1] [Such movement is often described as leaving a 'gap' behind (when the object is moved) and the moved or 'displaced' object is often referred to as the 'filler' for the gap.] Given that it is a critical empirical issue for language processing models to determine whether sentence interpretation is achieved via analysis of the relationships of the sentence *in their canonical order* (rather than in strict surface order), it is important to determine whether comprehension does indeed involve the active recovery of the *underlying* S–V–O order from the surface arrangement of the sentential elements. That is, are the out-of-order constituents (in this case, the direct object 'waitress') mentally reordered into their canonical position (following the verb) during comprehension? Currently, there exist a number of pieces of evidence in the sentence processing literature to support the notion that this does, indeed, occur (see e.g. Bever and McElree, 1988; Nicol and Swinney, 1989; Garnsey, Tanenhaus and Chapman, 1989); this chapter will provide considerably more detail in this regard.

There are two basic issues concerning how the comprehension device might recover the underlying relationship between discontinuous dependencies: *when* during ongoing comprehension the link between discontinuous elements (e.g. verb and direct object) is made and *how* this process takes place.

We will first consider some of the logical possibilities for the question of *when* the linkage takes place: if the process is a structurally principled one (i.e. if it is a comprehension procedure that occurs at structurally relevant processing points), then it should occur either as soon as a direct object is discovered to be missing following a verb (i.e. immediately after processing the verb) or at some later structural processing location (e.g. the end of the clause or sentence containing the dependency relationship, or after a first-pass parse is completed). If, on the other hand, the process is structurally unprincipled (i.e. such as would be found in a generic constraint satisfaction, or probabilistic cue-driven, or frequency-driven or associationistically driven account, e.g. Bates and MacWhinney, 1987; MacDonald, Pearlmutter and Seidenberg,1994), then linkage of the direct object with its verb should take place only when sufficient cues have been accumulated during comprehension to allow appropriate prediction of the nature of relevant linkage. In these models, such linkage will occur at (highly) varying points during processing, based on strength of the frequencies or cues available in each different sentence – but it will specifically *not* always occur 'immediately' (or at any *single* structurally principled processing point) in the sentence.

The issue of *how* processes linking the direct object (often called the 'filler') to the 'gap' after the verb might work also allows for several logical possibilities. For example, the linking of the verb to its object may take the form of an antecedent-directed search for a gap (a search initiated by discovery of a potential antecedent as marked by occurrence of the relativizer 'who' in the object-relative construction (see, sentence 2, above). Hence, when a relative pronoun occurs, it may signal to the comprehension system that the noun phrase (NP) it refers to will 'fill' a gap (following some verb) later in the sentence. If this were how the system processes such constructions, one might expect that the NP preceding the relative pronoun would be activated and *would maintain its activation* until a 'gap' is found. This hypothesis for linking discontinuous dependencies is known as the 'filler-driven' model (Frazier and Flores-d'Arcais, 1989). Alternatively, the linkage occurring in this dependency construction could be 'verb-driven'; whenever a verb which requires a direct object is encountered, and no direct object is found immediately following the verb, a search could be initiated over prior sentential material for a 'missing' constituent, resulting in 'reactivation' of the direct object when it is found. The key to deciding if the process which links a verb and its (displaced) direct object is 'verb-driven' or 'antecedent-driven', will be to determine if there is *re*activation of the antecedent at the gap position rather than *continued* activation. Additionally, of course, details about how the link is established will involve the resolution of a number of other issues such as: whether the search of an antecedent filler occurs serially or in parallel over possible antecedents, whether it is made over deep or over surface representations of the sentence, and whether it is guided by syntactic information (e.g. structural knowledge concerning which prior NPs are possible antecedent 'fillers' for the gap), or by prosodic information, or by probabilistic preferences. And, finally, the question of whether this process is an autonomous one is of critical knowledge in building any model of structural comprehension. All of these issues will be examined below.

Note that, very similarly to the issues we have outlined above concerning 'when' and 'how' discontinuous structural elements are linked, the same general issues exist for the connection between pronouns and their antecedents. That is, fundamental to our understanding of the comprehension process are answers to critical questions concerning *when* a search for an antecedent is initiated by the appearance of a pronoun (e.g. immediately, or at the end of the current clause) and *how* that search takes place (whether an initial candidate set is established that includes all previously mentioned nouns, or only those which are grammatically legal).

In the work that follows, we briefly review old (and report new) evidence which supports the view that, for non-brain-damaged adult listeners, the processes involved in comprehending both co-referential (pronominal) and purely structural discontinuous dependencies both appear to involve structurally principled and relatively immediate linkage of dependent elements. The two types of process do differ, however, as will be briefly touched on below.

Methodology and the study of language processing

A wide variety of experimental paradigms have been employed throughout the history of the study of language comprehension. These methods can be roughly divided into two types: 'off-line' and 'on-line' approaches. Off-line methods have proven useful in determining the general (or coarse-grained) characteristics of the comprehension process. Off-line methods are called 'off-line' because they evaluate language comprehension only *after* it has actually taken place. They typically involve untimed measures which standardly encourage the incorporation of everything the listener knows (world knowledge etc.) into a subject's response, and routinely involve conscious evaluation of the process being studied (some standard 'off-line' tasks are: sentence–picture matching, paraphrase, sentence recall). Such off-line methods, taking place as they do after comprehension has occurred, often miss rapid, non-consciously available details of how the comprehension actually took place; data from such tasks are often termed 'post-perceptual' data. In contrast, on-line methodologies are concerned with detailing information as it unfolds during ongoing sentence processing. On-line methods capture the moment-by-moment operations of the extremely rapid, unconscious, processes that underlie ongoing language comprehension. It is these 'on-line' techniques that will allow us to establish fine-grain models of language understanding. In this chapter we will focus on evidence from 'on-line' methodologies.

A number of 'on-line' methodologies are currently in use. Although many of these methodologies each have revealed important properties of language processing, cross-modal lexical priming (Swinney, Onifer, Prather and Hirshkowitz, 1979) has proven to be a particularly illuminative and sensitive measure of moment-by-moment sentence processing. Cross-modal lexical priming (CMLP) techniques come in many varieties, but all involve the following conditions and properties. First, the language material is presented auditorily to listeners, who are told that their major job is to understand the sentence(s) or discourse they hear. Listeners (experimental subjects) are tested for their comprehension of these materials at various points throughout the experiment, to keep their attention on the primary task of comprehension. Subjects also have a second task to perform while they are listening to and comprehending the auditory material: they are told that at some point a visual item will appear on a screen in front of them and they will have to make a decision about that visual item. This visual item may be a letter string [to which subjects may, for example, be required to make a lexical decision (word or not), a classifying decision (e.g. edible or not), or a 'naming' response] or, the visual item may be a picture (to which some type of classifying response is made, such as 'edible/non-edible'). Extensive work with the CMLP technique has shown that most two-choice classification responses work quite well in obtaining basic effects. Finally, we use evidence of 'priming' between material in the sentence and the response made to the visual target as a measure of what aspect of the auditory sentential material is being processed. Specifically, there is a planned relation between visual target classification on some of the trials (never more than 25% of all trials) and material in the sentence/discourse that is heard. On experimental trials the visual target (picture or word) is associatively/semantically related to a critical word or constituent that we are interested in studying in the sentence. Following the principle of automatic semantic priming, the occurrence of an auditory word (a 'prime') in the sentence just prior to the processing of an associatively or semantically related visual item results in speeded processing/classification of the visual target, a process termed 'priming' (see e.g. Meyer, Schvaneveldt and Ruddy, 1975; Neely, 1991).

There are several aspects of this technique that we wish to stress. To begin with, presentation of auditory discourse/sentential material *always* continues to the sentence's end; it is never stopped or modified, even when the visual probe/target is presented. Additionally, the visual target never occurs at the end of the sentence. This prevents the visual target from being integrated into the ongoing sentential material (provided, of course, that the sentential material is presented at normal volume levels and speed – see further discussion by Nicol, Swinney, Love and Hald, 1997; Swinney, Nicol, Love and Hald, 1998). Secondly, judgments about the visual targets never involve subjects making metalinguistic judgments about anything in the auditory material they hear (e.g. Was the word 'waitress' in the sentence?). This prevents metalinguistic examination of the auditory sentence, processing which involves conscious (non-automatic) processes in addition to normal comprehension processes (again, see Swinney, Nicol, Love and Hald, 1998; Shapiro, Swinney and Borsky, 1998, for more details). Finally, processing of the sentence is uninterrupted and 'normal', at least up to the point where the visual target is presented — *which is the final processing point we ever examine*. In this regard, the task differs considerably from most other on-line tasks which often ask the subject to evaluate each word in a sentence as it appears, or to hold a target in mind while the sentence is being processed. Thus, the CMLP task is one of the most sensitive, least intrusive behavioural techniques we have for the 'on-line' examination of the normal comprehension process.

The way in which this task is used in the two conditions of discontinuous dependency processing we are concerned with in this chapter can be seen in the two following examples.

3. Overt co-reference: (pronoun)
   The skier told the plumber that the doctor would * blame *him* * for the injury.

4. Structural dependency: (object-relative construction)
   The policeman saw the boy who the crowd at the party * accused * of the crime.

In sentence (3), visual target words related associatively to each of the three prior NPs in the sentence (skier, plumber, doctor) can be presented at each of the points during the sentence as indicated by the asterisk (*). In addition, control target words are presented at each of these points.[2] (Note that no subject hears a sentence more than once or sees more than one visual target word with that sentence.) Similarly, in sentence (4), visual targets related to various NPs in the sentence that are potentially the correct 'direct objects' can be presented at the points indicated by asterisks. In all cases, the first such point of presentation is a 'baseline' point — one in which residual activation for each of the NPs can be measured. The second such point always occurs at a theoretically relevant processing point in the sentence: for instance, in the example (3), it is just after the pronoun, so that the *'immediate* reactivation' hypothesis can be tested; in example (4), it is immediately after the verb, so that the immediate, verb-driven hypothesis can be tested. Obviously, target words can occur at any other theoretically relevant points during the sentence, to test for activation (or reactivation) of appropriate NPs during putative linking operations. In short, via the use of CMLP, we are exploiting the fact of priming to provide a basis for an existence proof about the time course of mental activation of some 'key' word in the sentence – in this case the antecedent filler for a structural gap.[3] The CMLP task allows us to know precisely when an item that must be linked in a dependency relationship later in the sentence is active during structural processing (and, when it is not). Further, it allows us to examine the time-course of activation of processing of all potential filler NPs (in structurally appropriate vs. structurally inappropriate positions, thereby allowing for examination of the role of structural knowledge on this process).

In what follows, we present information utilizing CMLP to detail the time-course of information integration and activation during the processing of both types of discontinuous dependencies in non-brain-damaged adults.

The processing of overt anaphors (pro-forms) in non-brain-damaged adults

The fundamental questions we will examine briefly in this section concern *when* and *how* the processor links reference-seeking elements (pronouns or reflexives) to their antecedents. Early research in this area suggested that these overt anaphors are more-or-less *immediately* linked to the antecedent NP to which they refer (see e.g. Corbett and Chang, 1983; Bever and McElree, 1988; Tanenhaus, Carlson and Seidenberg, 1985; Tanenhaus, Stowe and Carlson, 1985; see, however, Caramazza, Grober, Garvey and Yates, 1977). Although these studies demonstrated this apparent 'fact' via somewhat different methodologies, a number of the more influential of these investigations employed an end-of-the-sentence probe verification task in their work (the exception to this is Tanenhaus, Stowe and Carlson, 1985 who used a word-by-word reading task). One problem in interpreting these end-of-sentence probe studies is that the measures they use are taken temporally *after* the event of interest, thus confounding the results with 'off-line' factors such as conscious rumination, etc. Further, the time at which 'linkage' takes place during processing of the sentence obviously cannot be readily specified with this task. For this reason (and the others stated above) much of the more recent behavioural work in this field has involved the use of 'on-line' tasks such as CMLP.

Nicol (1988), for example, utilized CMLP to examine the reactivation of antecedents to both pronouns and reflexives during ongoing processing, employing sentences such as:

5. The swimmer told the skier that the doctor for the team was sure to blame *him* for the accident.
6. The swimmer told the skier that the doctor for the team was sure to blame *himself* for the accident.

Nicol (1988) found that for sentences such as (5), both 'swimmer' and 'skier' (all of the structurally permissible antecedents) were activated (primed relative to their controls) *immediately* after the pronoun occurred, whereas only the structurally correct antecedent, 'doctor' was reactivated after the reflexive in sentences such as (6). Thus, by utilizing these essentially identical sentences which differ only in terms of the pro-form employed (which makes them subject to different structural constraints governing reference), Nicol determined that: (1) only *syntactically legal antecedents* are reactivated (linked) to pro-forms during ongoing comprehension and that (2) this linkage occurs *immediately* upon encountering the pro-form in the sentence. This evidence, then, substantiates inferences from the earlier off-line work, and provides an initial indication of how certain discontinuous dependencies are processed 'on-line'.

The processing of structural dependencies by non-brain-damaged adults

A series of studies utilizing the CMLP technique (begun in 1982) have examined the linkage of the 'moved' direct object in object-relative constructions to its canonical position (following the verb) in sentences.

The first of these studies was undertaken in 1982 by Ford, Frauenfelder, Bresnan and Swinney and first reported in Swinney, Ford, Frauenfelder and Bresnan, 1987 (and referred to again in Nicol and Swinney, 1989). This study examined the processing of object-relative constructions such as in sentence (3) above (and repeated here):

The policeman saw the boy who the crowd at the party *[1] accused *[2] of the crime

At each test point, activation for the three first nouns in the sentence was examined at points both before and after the verb (at the baseline and gap positions, respectively). Thus, for this example, words related to: 'policeman', 'boy' and 'crowd' were presented at each of the two test points (as were unrelated control words) in a completely counterbalanced design. The results are easily described: at test point *[1] (the 'baseline' position) there was significant priming found for visual target words related to the last noun (e.g. 'crowd'), but there was no significant priming for words related to either the first noun (e.g. 'policeman') or the second noun (e.g. 'boy'). However, at test point *[2] (at the point of the gap – the structural dependency) there was significant priming *only* for the visual target related to 'boy' (the correct filler) but not for targets related to either 'policeman' or 'crowd'. Finally, there was a significant interaction between the factors of test point (*[1] vs. *[2]) and target type (related vs. control – priming) for the word 'boy' (see Table 3.1 for details).

Table 3.1. Priming scores in ms (lexical decision reaction times to control minus semantically related word) for each potential referent, at each probe point

Referent	Probe point	
	1	2
Boy	12_{ns}	27*
Crowd	44*	19_{ns}

* indicates significance at $p < 0.05$ in tests of *a priori* planned paired-comparisons (*t*-tests).

Several conclusions follow from this initial study. First, reactivation of the appropriate antecedent for a structural gap occurs *immediately* – as soon as it is discovered there is no direct object following the verb. This result is in keeping with results from other methodological techniques such as reading times at potential gap sites (e.g. Crain and Fodor, 1985; Stowe, 1986) and Evoked Potential measures (e.g. Garnsey, Tanenhaus and Chapman, 1989) which also support the conclusion that once a verb which requires a direct object is encountered (and no direct object is found), a search for a prior-occurring direct object is undertaken immedi-

ately, resulting in *re*activation of that NP. Further, these results suggest that
the search for the direct object is not performed at random or in a way that
reactivates all previous NPs; rather, *only* the actual (correct) filler is reactivated. Thus, the link between a verb and its displaced direct object is
guided by structural knowledge. For example, such knowledge dictates
that the missing direct object can *not* be the subject of the verb for which it
is also a direct object (e.g. the word 'crowd'; no priming was found for the
target related to 'crowd' at the test point following the verb). Note that
there was no priming for a target related to the appropriate antecedent
filler for the gap ('boy') at the test point prior to the gap (the baseline).
Thus, it appears that the process which establishes a link between a gap
and its antecedent/direct object is *verb-driven* (in that the direct object is
not activated and then kept active until a verb is found, but, rather, it is
reactivated after the verb is understood). In short, this early study strongly
suggested that the connection between a filler and a structural gap was an
immediate, structurally driven, automatic process in comprehension.

A number of subsequent studies utilizing the CMLP technique have
been performed which provide more detail about the nature of this
process. For example, Love and Swinney, 1996, examined a large number
of temporally distributed test points during comprehension to obtain
more detail about the time course of reactivation of such direct-object
antecedents during comprehension. They also examined whether the
search for antecedents was conducted over a surface structure form of the
sentence, or over a 'deeper' sentential representation. To do this, they
utilized lexical ambiguities as direct objects in object-relative constructions. The reasoning behind this study is based on the well-established
findings that all meanings of a lexically ambiguous word are initially
activated when the word is heard (e.g. Swinney, 1979; Tanenhaus, Leiman
and Seidenberg, 1979). Thus, if all meanings of the ambiguous direct
object (filler) are found to be *re*activated at the gap position following the
verb, an argument could be sustained that the search for an antecedent
filler occurs over a surface (acoustic) representation of the sentence.
However, if only the 'contextually appropriate meaning' of the antecedent
direct-object ambiguity is reactivated after the verb, then the search for the
antecedent must be over a 'deeper' representation of the sentence – one
in which a single meaning for the ambiguous word has been determined
and stored.[4] Subjects were presented (auditorily) with sentences such as:

7. The professor insisted that the exam be completed in ink, so Jimmy
   used the new *pen*[*1] that his mother-in-law recently[*2] purchased[*3] _
   because the multiple colours allowed for more creativity.

Priming for each meaning of the filler 'pen' (i.e. 'pencil' and 'jail') was
examined at each of three target presentation points (marked by *).
Significant priming for both meanings of the ambiguity (the primary, most

frequent meaning – 'pencil' and the secondary, less frequent meaning-'jail') occured at test point #1 – immediately following initial occurrence of the ambiguity in the sentence. (This provided yet another demonstration of exhaustive access of word meanings for lexical ambiguities in biasing contexts).[5] At test point #2 (prior to the critical verb, but after the initial occurrence of the antecedent direct object), no significant priming was found for either the primary or secondary meaning of the ambiguity. Finally, at the critical test point #3 (immediately following the verb), a significant priming effect was found for just the primary (and contextually relevant) meaning of the ambiguity; there was no significant priming for the secondary meaning of the antecedent direct object. The interaction between the non-significant effect at test point #2 and the significant effect for the primary meaning of the direct object at test point #3 was itself significant, indicating that only the primary meaning of the ambiguity was significantly *re*activated at the gap.

This study found reactivation rather than continued activation for the filler, and hence supported the verb-driven account that what triggers reactivation of the filler is the failure to find an object after a verb which requires an object. Furthermore, this study demonstrated that the search for the direct object takes place via a deep, non-surface, representation of the sentence (because only one meaning of the ambiguity was reactivated, rather than all meanings).

In a related study, the effect of plausibility in 'guiding' this linkage of the verb and direct object in object-relative constructions has been initially examined, with a goal of examining issues concerning the modularity of this process (i.e. the independence of this structurally driven process from world knowledge). In this study, subjects heard sentences such as:

8a. Everyone watched the enormous heavyweight boxer that the small 12-year-old boy on the corner had*[1] hugged*[2] _so intensely.
8b. Everyone watched the enormous heavyweight boxer that the small 12-year-old boy on the corner had*[1] beaten*[2] _so brutally.

The NP 'the enormous heavyweight boxer' is a plausible direct object of the verb 'hugged' in 8a but it is *not* a plausible direct object for the verb 'beaten' in 8b. It is, however, the structurally correct antecedent filler (object) in both cases. In both sentence types significant priming was obtained for target probes related to 'boxer', but not for those related to 'boy' immediately after the verb. Thus, these results support the view that the linkage between the verb and displaced direct object, although structurally driven, is independent from top-down knowledge/plausibility information. Hence the process is putatively a modular one.

Finally, from recent work (Swinney and Love, 1998) we know that the rate of processing (the speed at which the speech arrives to the listener) considerably changes the parameters of this reactivation process – thus implicating factors of memory and automaticity in the recovery of structurally based discontinuous dependencies.

Thus, we know that the processing of discontinuous dependency relationships is driven by a need to recover an underlying, canonical order of perceptual/sentential elements during ongoing comprehension. The process is triggered by the discovery of an 'incomplete' structural relationship in the surface form of the sentence – i.e. a verb which requires a direct object, where no direct object is found following the verb. The process by which the verb is linked to the direct object involves the search of a non-superficial, meaning-based representation of the sentence. That search is initiated immediately (not at the end of the sentence, but immediately once the direct object is detected as missing), and it is structurally driven. Finally, the search is neither changed nor directed by semantic/world knowledge/plausibility, but it is considerably affected by rate-of-speech.

The processing of overt anaphors (pro-forms) in brain-damaged adults

The remainder of this chapter will focus on what information can be gained by exploring the on-line processing of people who have sustained unilateral damage to localized areas of the brain. These brain damage populations serve as a unique resource to examine the neural architecture of the brain with respect to language function.

It is widely accepted that differential damage to particular areas of the left hemisphere (and typically not the right) causes language impairments (aphasia) in most right-handers. (However, there has been much debate about the issue of the localizability of language within the left hemisphere, and about whether or not the right hemisphere has any language capacity at all.)

The results from off-line unconstrained assessment of language and classic standardized testing measures (e.g. Boston Diagnostic Aphasia Examination, Goodglass and Kaplan, 1972b) have discriminated a number of major groups of language impairment within the brain-damaged population. Two groups in particular have been of special interest: those who appeared to have overt production deficits with relatively spared comprehension (Broca's aphasic patients) and those who displayed the opposite patterns of behavioural deficits – fluent speech production with impaired comprehension (Wernicke's aphasic patients).[6] It was discovered that these distinctions did not actually hold when a careful investigation of the language abilities was performed (Caramazza and Zurif, 1976). In fact, via sentence–picture matching tests, it was discovered that those patients classified as Broca's aphasic patients displayed distinct comprehension problems in addition to their production deficits.

In investigating the role(s) of particular neural regions in real-time language comprehension, a number of studies employing the cross-modal priming paradigm have been conducted. The studies described below investigate the processing of both antecedent-pronoun and filler-gap dependencies.

Work that is currently in progress looking at the processing of overt pronouns and reflexives during sentence processing strongly suggests, at least with respect to language processing, that there are differential roles of the neural substrates underlying the two aphasias. In this CMLP study, three Broca's, three Wernicke's, and two right hemisphere damaged control patients were presented with sentences that contained either a pronoun or reflexive (modified from Nicol, 1988) such as (9).

9. The boxer$_i$ said that the skier$_j$ in the hospital had blamed *him$_i$/self$_j$* for the recent injury.

In addition, they were presented with visual probe words which either were semantically related to the second NP (*skier* in example above) or were unrelated control words.[7] The results for the Wernicke's aphasics and unilateral right hemisphere damaged (control) patients are very straightforward: at the offset of the reflexive (*himself*) there is significant facilitation for words related to *skier* (the structurally-appropriate antecedent), but at the offset of the pronoun, there was no such facilitation for words related to *skier*. (Right hemisphere patients: 92 ms priming effect for the reflexive condition and 11 ms effect for the pronoun condition; Wernicke's aphasic patients: a significant priming effect of 44 ms for the reflexive condition and a non-significant priming effect of 10 ms for the pronoun condition.) The Broca's aphasic patients, on the other hand, demonstrate a very different (aberrant) pattern of effects: significant facilitation for words related to *skier*, after processing the *pronoun* (69 ms priming effect) and a non-significant effect of 9 ms for the *reflexive* condition. Here the normal structurally guided co-referential reflex is clearly disrupted, suggesting that the neural region typically involved in Broca's aphasia plays a critical role in the automatic routines underlying coreference during auditory sentence comprehension.

This dissociation in processing extends to other types of constructions as well. In investigating subject relative clause constructions, Zurif, Swinney, Prather, Solomon and Bushell (1993) presented sentences such as 'The man liked the tailor$_i$ with the British accent *[1] who$_i$ *[2] claimed to know the queen'. In this sentence, there is a co-referential link between *the tailor* and the relative pronoun *who*.[8] As seen in Table 3.2, results from this study with Broca's and Wernicke's aphasic patients revealed a striking dissociation: Wernicke's aphasic patients displayed 'normal' processing (reactivation of antecedent at the point of the relative pronoun) with no evidence of activation at the baseline position, and Broca's aphasic patients displayed an aberrant pattern of processing at the point of the pronoun (no priming for the correct antecedent).

Table 3.2. Priming effects (in ms control minus experimental) for subject relative constructions for both Broca's and Wernicke's aphasic patients at both the baseline (prior to relative pronoun) and 'gap' (following the relative pronoun) position.

	Baseline (*1)	Following relative pronoun (*2)
Wernicke's	+44	+125*
Broca's	−20	−68

*$p < 0.03$.

The processing of discontinuous structural dependencies in brain-damaged adults

Swinney, Zurif, Prather and Love (1996) found the same pattern of results obtained with these populations for object-relative clauses as they did for the pro-form and subject relative cases just described above. They presented Broca's and Wernicke's aphasic patients with sentences such as 'The priest enjoyed the drink$_i$ that the caterer was *[1] serving t$_i$ *[2] to the guests.' Again, using the CMLP paradigm, they found evidence for reactivation of the antecedent at the gap (*[2]) for Wernicke's aphasic patients but not for Broca's aphasic patients [again, with no priming at a baseline position (*[1]), hence reactivation occurred] (see Table 3.3).

Table 3.3. Priming effects (in ms) for control minus experimental relative constructions for both Broca's and Wernicke's aphasic populations at both baseline (pre-verb) and gap (post-verb) positions

	Baseline (control minus experimental)	Following verb (control minus experimental)
Wernicke's	+3	+108*
Broca's	+122	−9

*$p < 0.02$.

   Taken together, these findings suggest that the area of the brain affected by Broca's aphasia is crucial for the automatic reflexes responsible for rapidly establishing links among sentence elements consistent with the time constraints on sentence processing. In contrast, the Wernicke's aphasics showed no impairment in the automatic processes involved in such computations. However, they do typically show robust impairments in overall comprehension. Therefore, the region implicated in Wernicke's area may be involved in later-acting processes, such as integration of whole-sentence information or the computation of sentence-level meaning.

Acknowledgements

The authors gratefully acknowledge support from NIH DC02984, NIH DC00494 and NIDCD DC01409 for the research reported in this chapter and the National Center for Neurogenic Communication Disorders at the University of Arizona for supporting the writing of this chapter.

Notes

[1] This concept comes principally from formal linguistic theories in which underlying thematic/semantic relationships (meaning) are treated as a constant that is maintained regardless of the superficial form of the sentence (transformational and related linguistic approaches); hence the distinction between deep and surface structure in Generative Transformation Grammar, Chomsky (1965); see also Government and Binding Theory, Chomsky (1981).

[2] Note that all effects are evaluated in comparison to lexical decision reaction time to a 'control letter string' presented at each of these test points; a 'control letter string' is a word that is associatively/semantically *un*related to the key word in the sentence, but which is matched to the 'experimental' (related) letter string on the basis of *a priori* reaction time (lexical decisions taken on the words presented in isolation).

[3] McKoon and Ratcliff,1994 (see also McKoon, Ratcliff and Albritton, 1996) have presented arguments in which they have suggested that use of the CMLP technique for examining structural processing contains a confound – namely that the 'visual experimental target words constitute better 'continuation' (or, a better 'fit with') the ongoing sentence than do the 'control' target words. Thus, they claim that priming found in these studies is an effect caused by the 'goodness-of-fit' of probes into the sentence, and not by 'reactivation' or 'continued activation' of the filler. For the record, the single example McKoon and Ratcliff discuss *did* have such a confound. However, in all other studies (including those presented here) the experimental and control probes have been equated for all types of 'goodness-of-fit' at each probe point, and hence *no* such confound exists for any of these results, thus invalidating McKoon and Ratcliff's claims. In short, the CMLP task is a sensitive and unconfounded measure of lexical activations during structural processing. See Swinney, Nicol, Love and Hald (1998), as well as Nicol, Swinney, Love and Hald (1997) and Walenski (1997), for further discussion of this and related issues.

[4] This study also controlled precisely for various potential confounds in the original CMLP study on this phenomenon; see e.g. McKoon and Ratcliff (1994) and Nicol, Fodor and Swinney (1994).

[5] We note in passing that strong biasing contexts which exactly replicated the Tabossi (1988) criteria were employed in this study, but they had no effect on lexical access – again strongly supporting the claim of initial contextual independence for lexical access.

[6] The aphasia classifications are named after the neurologists who discovered the neuroanatomical link to the particular behavioral deficit (Broca in 1861 and Wernicke in 1874). Broca's area is located in the third frontal convolution of the left hemisphere (Brodmann 44). Wernicke's area is located in the posterior regions of the left hemisphere, superior temporal gyrus (Brodmann 22).

[7] Based on the existing evidence in the literature for an automatic linking of the antecedent and the co-referent (Nicol, 1988; Fodor, 1989 to name two), this study was simplified so as to only test for one of the noun phrases – in particular, the second

noun phrase (the correct antecedent for the reflexive). Moreover, again for design simplicity, only the offset of the overt anaphor was tested.

[8.] We note here that although this is a case of co-reference involving a relative *pronoun*, it is also a potential case of a structural dependency – created by the putative movement of the subject from the position now occupied by the relative pronoun. Hence it bridges the co-reference and structural-dependency cases.

Chapter 4
Semantic composition: Processing parameters and neuroanatomical considerations

EDGAR B. ZURIF AND MARIA M. PIÑANGO

Introduction

In this chapter, we first provide a perspective on the interface between syntactic and conceptual representations. This is the stage at which arrangements of nouns, verbs, adjectives and the like are brought into correspondence with lexical information about objects, events, properties, times and quantities. We then isolate an operation that mediates this correspondence. Finally, we suggest the neuroanatomical underpinnings of this operation.

The syntactic–semantic interface: some general considerations

In many instances of sentence interpretation, the way in which word meanings are combined is straightforwardly a function of the way in which the words are combined in syntactic structure. Consider the sentence, 'The girl snoozed for a long time after the grown-ups had left'. 'The girl' (subject) is performing an activity, 'snooze', for the period of time indicated by the phrase, 'for a long time'. Here, syntax establishes the structural relations among the words of the sentence and the meanings of those words are simply mapped on to this structure in a one-to-one fashion. Composition can be said to be syntactically transparent.

By contrast, consider the sentence, 'The girl twitched for a long time after the grown-ups had left'. Our understanding of this sentence requires that we paste in an extra bit of meaning. The interpretation we retrieve is that the girl twitched *repeatedly*, and this is not signalled by any obvious morpho-syntactic element. In effect, our interpretation of this sentence is not syntactically transparent. Yet, this phenomenon, which is termed aspectual coercion (Moens and Steedman, 1987; Pustejovsky, 1991, 1995;

Jackendoff, 1997), and is in Jackendoff's (1997) words a form of 'enriched composition', arises unavoidably and must somehow be explained.[1]

One possible way to account for aspectual coercion is to do so syntactically, viz. by providing a functional category for 'repetition'. In this account, a repetition node is positioned on a syntactic tree to confer a repetition feature for the verb, just as tense and agreement nodes confer tense and agreement features.

This solution is unsatisfactory, however. There would have to be quite a lot of different syntactic nodes of this general sort. The fact is that there are quite a few circumstances requiring the incorporation of extra semantic material in the interpretation of a constituent – circumstances that have nothing to do with repetition (and indeed, seem to resist any kind of syntactic patch). One such case involves verbs like 'begin', 'enjoy' and 'try' which semantically imply a process being begun, enjoyed or tried and which, when they occur with a direct object that is not a process, require the insertion of extra material to achieve semantic well-formedness. So, for instance, 'Bill began the book' needs the insertion of 'to read' or 'to write' for the sentence to make sense (Pustejovsky, 1995; Jackendoff, 1997). And there are cases of a quite different sort such as mass nouns appearing as count nouns and count nouns, as mass nouns – respectively, 'I'll have three coffees' and 'We're having octopus for dinner' in which the semantic information expressed by 'portion of' and 'meat' must be added to the sentence meanings for the count/mass and mass/count transitions to take place. And these cases of enriched composition hardly cover the wide range of phenomena already isolated. (See Jackendoff (1997) for a full discussion.)

Our data will provide another reason for rejecting a syntactic explanation for the addition of a repetition function to such sentences as 'The girl twitched for a long time...'. We will show that the operation that adds this information is slower acting than are reflexive syntactic operations – that it seems, instead, to occur within a time frame reserved for semantic operations. We will return to this point.

Yet, even if aspectual coercion is not a syntactically based phenomenon, several researchers have still sought to explain it within the GB/Minimalist tradition – i.e. within a system in which the correspondence between syntax and semantics is always syntactically transparent. One way to maintain this feature is, quite simply, by positing multiple senses of a word. So, for our earlier example of aspectual coercion, there would be two lexical entries for 'twitch' – one for 'twitch one time only' and another for 'twitch repeatedly'. This type of account, however, overlooks the fact that adding 'repetition' to the meaning of a sentence is an unavoidable consequence of the combination of any verb glossing an agentive, reversible, bounded activity (e.g. dive, jump, strike, slap...) and any type of bounding phrase (e.g. 'for an hour', 'for some time', 'until the cows come home'...). At the very least then, attempting to account for aspectual coercion as a lexical idiosyncracy just misses a generalization. And this approach becomes even more tortuous and ad hoc upon consideration of the other, varied circumstances demanding the pasting in of extra meaning (enriched composition).

There is another way to maintain the GB/Minimalist framework, however. This is by incorporating truth-conditional interpretation operations. Thus, in the GB/Minimalist framework, syntax delivers a Logical Form which, in turn, is the input to truth-conditional interpretation; and at this level, triggered by 'type' mismatches, a set of shifting/coercion mechanisms add the extra meaning (Partee and Rooth, 1983; Chierchia, 1984; Klein and Sag, 1985). This notion of type shifting has been incorporated by Pustejovsky (1995) into his sweeping proposal of a generative lexical system. In Pustejovsky's system, lexical items with detailed internal structures dynamically generate different senses when combined with one another in phrases and sentences.

There is yet another account of aspectual coercion – this due to the work of Jackendoff (1997). It constitutes a radical departure from the syntactocentric architecture of the GB/Minimalist tradition. Building partly on Pustejovsky's (1991, 1995) account, Jackendoff proposes a system comprised, in part, of syntactic and conceptual structures in which *both* components are generative – not just the syntactic one. This arrangement enables meaning to be generated even if not found in the lexical conceptual structures of items composing a sentence. Thus, Jackendoff (1997) accounts for aspectual coercion by interpolating a coercion function (that is, a piece of meaning, 'repetition') between the verb and the otherwise unsuitable temporal expression.

Even though these last mentioned accounts differ on how best to capture aspectual coercion – whether by lexical means or by function interpolation at the syntactic–semantic interface – they agree on its being a compositional semantic phenomenon – a form of enriched composition – rooted to some kind of non-syntactic *combinational* operation. And our work has sought to characterize this operation – to determine whether it is isolable as comprehension unfolds in real time and also whether it is neuroanatomically identifiable. We will deal with these two concerns in turn.

Semantic composition in real time

Our analysis of aspectual coercion from a real-time perspective has relied on a dual-task interference paradigm. In particular, we used a cross-modal lexical decision version of this paradigm. The primary task here requires that a subject listen to and understand an auditorily presented sentence. The secondary task is a lexical decision task. It requires a subject to decide whether or not a letter string forms a word, the string being flashed on a computer screen while the subject is listening to the sentence. Crucially, when the string does form a word, it is unrelated to any word or idea in the sentence.

Our use of this paradigm carried with it a well-worn assumption: that the two tasks – listening to the sentence and making a lexical decision – compete for the same limited resources. And given this assumption, we hypothesized that a sentence requiring aspectual coercion, or enriched composition, would burden processing resources more than a sentence whose interpretation is syntactically transparent. In effect, we hypothesized that, like other semantic operations (Shapiro, Zurif and Grimshaw, 1987, 1989), the operation underlying coercion comes with a computational cost – a cost reflected by a longer reaction time in the secondary lexical decision task.

Even granting this nexus of possibilities, we still had to determine, roughly, where and for how long during comprehension the cost of aspectual coercion would be exacted. We could count on it being mandatory (in relevant contexts) and strictly local, operating over the verb phrase only. But the time frame of the operation was another matter.

Here we were guided by recent evidence that the formation of a semantic representation appears to follow a slower-developing, longer-lasting time course than do syntactic operations. Specifically, both Boland (1996) and McElree and Griffith (1995) have reported that syntactic violations are noticed faster than semantic violations. McElree and Griffith (1995) have charted this difference in great detail: using a speed–accuracy trade-off manipulation, they have shown that although syntactic violations are reliably detected after 230 ms, semantic violation are first reliably detected only after 279 ms. Because anomaly detection must be done on the basis of a previously formed representation, we figured that the semantic operation underlying aspectual coercion would be revealed at some point between 230 and 279 ms – that this brief period would provide a window in which the cost of a semantic operation could be observed in a relatively unobscured fashion. Accordingly, we positioned the secondary task 250 ms after coercion was licensed – a point that always appeared while the sentence was still being auditorily delivered.

Some additional details: we constructed pairs of experimental sentences, each pair containing one transparent sentence and one sentence requiring aspectual coercion (i.e. enriched composition). The two were identical except for the verb.

                         250 ms
                          ┌────────LEATHER
The little girl dogpaddled in the pool until the teacher told her to eat if she wanted to keep her strength up.

                         250 ms
                          ┌────────SILVER
The little girl dived in the pool until the teacher told her to eat if she wanted to keep her strength up.

The first sentence in this pair is interpretable in a syntactically transparent fashion. The second requires enriched composition. That is aspectual coercion must take place – the semantic content 'sequence' or 'repetition' must somehow be pasted in.

The letter-string probes constituting the secondary task are also shown in this example. We note in this respect that probe–sentence pairings (*leather* and *silver*)were counterbalanced for the experiment such that half the subjects saw the probe–sentence pairings depicted above and the other half saw reverse pairings. This, of course, guarded against any accidental advantages for particular sentence–probe combinations.

Two other controls also warrant mention. The first of these did away with word frequency confounds. The verbs glossing point action activities and thereby requiring aspectual coercion were always of equal or greater frequency than their syntactically transparent counterparts. So if a frequency advantage were to have influenced the data, it would have blunted the cost of the operation underlying aspectual coercion. The second control, the administration of a sentence plausibility questionnaire, ensured that the transparent sentences were neither more nor less plausible than those requiring coercion [see Piñango (1998) for complete details].

With all these controls in place, we set out to observe whether the operation underlying aspectual coercion is isolable in real time. And to state the outcome simply, *it is isolable* – lexical decision took significantly longer for letter strings paired with sentences requiring aspectual coercion (enriched composition) than for letter strings paired with syntactically transparent sentences. In effect, we discovered the real-time cost of a combinatorial semantic process.

Moreover, our data offer strong support for the argument that aspectual coercion depends upon a generative operation as opposed to one based on lexical polysemy. A notion of polysemy that could, in principle, account for our results would have to be that more polysemous verbs take more time to process than less polysemous ones. But as it happens, the reverse is true. A number of studies have shown that more polysemous words are easier to process than less polysemous ones; in effect they are less computationally costly – as measured by reaction time (Jastrzembski and Stanners, 1975; Jastrzembski, 1981; Gerratt and Jones, 1987; Kellas, Ferraro and Simpson, 1988; Millis and Button, 1989). Further, more polysemous words are on average of higher frequency than less polysemous words (Miller, 1985; Lee, 1990). And as we have already noted, because we wanted to rule out any simple frequency explanation for our results – an account whereby verbs requiring coercion were more costly to process because they were less frequent – these verbs were chosen to be either of equal or higher frequency than their 'transparent' counterparts. Because frequency, itself, decreases the cost of lexical activation, by rigging the frequencies the way we did, we also ruled out any potential polysemy-based explanation.

We are left then with a generative and computationally isolable operation that takes place as comprehension progresses. And these properties suggest to us that coercion exists not at some extra-sentential inferential level but at the level where syntactic and semantic structure meet.

The neuroanatomical underpinning of semantic composition

Our first attempt to discover the neuroanatomy of semantic composition (in the form of aspectual coercion) relies on the study of aphasia. This work is not far along; even so, we are beginning to see a contrast with what is known of the neuroanatomy of syntactic composition.

Our connection to neuroanatomy turns on the lesion localizing value of Broca's and Wernicke's aphasia. Thus, although there is considerable variation in lesion extent, particularly for Broca's aphasia, which is associated with large superficial and deep lesions, often including, but certainly not limited to the frontal operculum (Broca's area), the fact is that the modal lesion site for this form of aphasia is different from that for Wernicke's aphasia. For the latter, the greatest involvement appears to be inferior to the Sylvian fissure, implicating especially the auditory association cortex located in the posterior superior portion of the first temporal gyrus. (See, among others, Mohr, 1976; Vignolo, 1988; Alexander, Naeser and Palumbo, 1990; Goodglass, 1993; Dronkers, Wilkin, Van Valin, Redfern and Jaeger, 1994 for localization data.) Indeed, at least 80% of Broca's and Wernicke's aphasias appear accountable by lesions in these modal regions (Harold Goodglass and Marty Albert, personal communications, 1994).

Far more is known about the linguistic commitment of the brain region associated with Broca's aphasia. It has been established that this region is crucially involved in the construction of syntactic dependency relations – specifically, in the formation of antecedent-gap links. Further, as will be apparent from Swinney et al.'s chapter in this volume (Chapter 3), this brain region does not seem to be the locus of syntactic representations per se, but rather seems to play a processing role. It seems to provide the resources necessary for carrying out 'gap-filling' in real time – particularly for supporting the fast-acting, reflexive nature of this operation (e.g. Zurif and Swinney, 1994).[2]

This emphasis on timing is further legitimized by the fact that the left anterior lesions associated with Broca's aphasia do not seem to disrupt sentence processing at the semantic level. Broca's patients appear normally sensitive in real time to the argument-taking properties of verbs (Shapiro and Levine, 1990; Shapiro, Gordon, Hack and Killackey, 1993), and indeed, show no comprehension problems when the syntax is simple – just what would be expected given that semantic processing is temporally less demanding than syntactic processing (Swinney and Osterhout, 1990; McElree and Griffith, 1995; Boland, 1996). The point here is that a diminishment in processing speed sufficient to disrupt a syntactic operation need not also affect semantic operations.

We cannot over-emphasize the syndrome-specificity of this characterization – its applicability only to Broca's aphasia. In direct contrast to the Broca's region, the posterior brain region associated with Wernicke's aphasia does *not* seem crucial for the syntactic reflex of gap-filling (e.g. Zurif and Swinney, 1994). And whatever commitment it might have to other syntactic operations, it also plays an important semantic role (e.g. Shapiro and Levine, 1990; Shapiro et al., 1993) – again in contrast to the Broca's region.

However, most clinical and experimental observations of the Wernicke's patients' semantic impairment have been at the level of single words and this leaves unexplained aspects of their comprehension performance at the sentence level – in particular, their unpredictable variability at this level. In short, we know that the left posterior cortex is involved in semantic work, but we do not know how this involvement plays out at the sentence level. And it is this void that we have lately sought to fill.

Our first step has been to study aphasic comprehension *off-line* – that is, in terms of patterns of comprehension success and failure. In particular, we have been trying to determine if sentence comprehension in Wernicke's aphasia is affected in a manner that directly implicates the distinction between enriched and syntactically transparent composition. Our hypothesis guiding this first step is that the Wernicke's comprehension problem, but not the Broca's, will be particularly apparent in circumstances requiring aspectual coercion – indeed, we expect Broca's patients to have a sentence-comprehension problem only in the total absence of semantic constraints, not when more semantic work is required.

Like our first on-line study with neurologically intact subjects, our study of aphasic comprehension off-line has turned on aspectual coercion. Our task requires patients to answer a binary-choice question for each sentence presented. So, for example, for the sentence, 'The tiger jumped for an hour', we contrast 'Did the tiger jump only one time?' (the incorrect choice) vs. 'Did the tiger jump time and time again?' (the correct choice). Once again, this is an example of a sentence requiring enriched composition – the semantic content, 'repetition', must be generated. Its syntactically transparent counterpart is 'The tiger jumped over the tree', and again, the contrast is between 'Did the tiger jump only one time?' vs. 'Did the tiger jump time and time again?' Note that for this first effort, we chose only those verbs that signify activities that are precisely temporally bound or 'telic' (Pustejovsky, 1995). Accordingly, we contrast enriched vs. syntactically transparent composition by using the same verb placed in two different contexts. To be more specific, the material consisted of 16 verbs (chosen from our on-line study) each embedded in two sentences (as exemplified just above) for a total of 32 contrasts.

The procedure consisted of playing a sentence on tape, stopping the tape immediately after the sentence, posing the binary-choice question, and while asking the question, holding up one index finger to signify one alternative and the other index finger to signify the other alternative.

To date we have tested three Broca's and two Wernicke's patients. And the data support our hypothesis. None of the Broca's patients showed an important difference between the enriched and transparent conditions, averaging 14 correct out of 16 for the transparent condition (the individual scores were 12, 14 and 16), and 14.3 correct out of 16 for the enriched condition (the individual scores were 13, 14 and 16). We think that the few errors that were observed for the Broca's patients reflect the memory load imposed by our task – the requirement that information be held in memory while the tape was stopped and the binary choice question asked. But whatever the cause, it must be emphasized that the few errors were evenly distributed over the two conditions. By contrast, both Wernicke's patients did show a difference and in the predicted direction. For the syntactically transparent sentences, one scored 12 out of 16 correct and the other 14 out of 16. But for the enriched sentences they scored, respectively, only 8 out of 16 and 9 out of 16 correct. That is, on average they had more than twice the number of errors for enriched sentences than for transparent ones.

It is a slim database, but an encouraging one for our effort to make sense of the sentence comprehension performance of Wernicke's patients. More generally, it allows us (at least tentatively) to align a linguistically principled syntactic–semantic partition with a neuroanatomical distribution between anterior and posterior regions of the left hemisphere.

Acknowledgements

The writing of this chapter and the research reported in it were supported by NIH grants DC 02984, AG 10496 and DC 00081.

Notes

[1] The aspect we refer to here is 'situation' aspect – i.e., Aktionsarten. Situation aspect captures the temporal characteristics of a verb or a verb and its complement(s). This can be obseved in the contrast:
1a. Jane drew a circle (temporally bound, only one circle was drawn)
  b. Jane drew circles (temporally unbounded, there is no limit to the amount of circles that were drawn)
Situation aspect stands in contrast to viewpoint aspect which refers to the different perspectives a speaker can take with respect to the temporal course of development of an event or state. There are two types of viewpoint aspect: perfective,
2a. She drew a circle yesterday (speaker looks at the event as a whole) and imperfective:
  b. She was drawing a circle yesterday (speaker is looking at the event from the inside)
As noted, when we refer to aspectual coercion, the 'aspectual' part of it is restricted to situational aspect.
[2] It is worth while noting here that the PEI and fMRI analyses of normal comprehension are also beginning to identify the importance for syntactic processing of the cortical region implicated in Broca's aphasia (Stromswold, Caplan, Alpert and Rauch, 1996; Caplan, Alpert and Waters, 1998).

Chapter 5
Syntactic displacement in Broca's agrammatic aphasia

MARIA M. PIÑANGO

Introduction

It has by now been well established that the deficit observed in Broca's agrammatic comprehension at the sentence level lends itself to principled characterization. One example of this is found in the Trace Deletion Hypothesis (TDH) (Grodzinsky, 1990). The TDH describes the comprehension deficit observed in Broca's aphasia, roughly, as an inability to deal with syntactic displacement [see also Hickok, Zurif and Canseco-Gonzalez (1993) and Mauner, Fromkin and Cornell (1993) for different implementations of the same insight].

The aim of descriptive generalizations such as this is to capture a widely observed pattern of performance in Broca's comprehension where constructions such as the active (e.g. *The cat chased the dog*), subject relative (e.g. *The cat that chased the dog is big*) and subject cleft (e.g. *This is the cat that chased the dog*) are comprehended at a level greater than *chance*, and constructions such as the passive (e.g. *The dog was chased by the cat*), object relative (e.g. *The dog that the cat chased is big*) and object cleft (e.g. *This is the dog that the cat chased*) exhibit a performance level within the *chance* range.

Briefly, the TDH accounts for this pattern within the Government and Binding framework (Chomsky, 1981) by positing (1) that traces of moved arguments are deleted in the Broca's agrammatic representation,[1] and (2) that in case the first referential noun phrase of the sentence is left without a thematic role (due to trace deletion), the role of *agent* is assigned to it by default. Predictions for agrammatic comprehension follow from the interaction between an impaired representation (one that lacks argument traces) and the default (agent-first) strategy.

The necessity to incorporate an extra-linguistic element in the generalization, such as the *agent*-first strategy, is given by the fact that not all types of syntactic displacement result in impaired levels of performance. So, even though there is syntactic displacement in both subject and object relatives, *chance* performance surfaces only in object relatives. A similar situation arises in actives and passives and subject and object clefts where *chance* performance occurs only in object clefts and passives even though all four constructions are taken to involve some kind of argument displacement.

As it happens, in those constructions where *chance* performance has been observed (object relatives/object clefts and passives) syntactic displacement takes place in the form of *movement from object position*. This kind of displacement, in turn, reverses the canonical order of thematic roles licensed by the verb (i.e. the undergoer or recipient of the action appears in the sentence before the actor or causer of the action). This suggests that even though the evidence for Broca's agrammatic comprehension allows a movement-based characterization, it does not distinguish movement itself from one of its possible consequences – deviation from canonical order of thematic roles in surface representation. Here, I will pursue the notion that it is presence or absence of canonicity in syntactic representation and not syntactic displacement that is central to the problem of Broca's agrammatic comprehension.[2]

The question that follows from this notion is, then, what kind of linguistic mechanism can be damaged in Broca's aphasia such that deviation from canonical order could trigger impaired comprehension? This is the focus of the following section.

The Argument Linking Hypothesis

Suppose that the language system has two linking mechanisms that can potentially establish correspondence between arguments in semantic structure and syntactic representation (that is, mechanisms that tell the system whether a semantic relation 'argument of' can be connected to a given syntactic relation such as 'subject of'). One mechanism, *semantic linking*, is purely semantically based and establishes correspondence between arguments and *linear positions* in the sentence (first, second, etc...). The other is *syntactic linking* which establishes correspondence between arguments and *syntactic functions* based on syntactic principles.

Semantic linking embodies the intuition, present in all descriptions of Broca's comprehension I know and in more flushed-out theories of language representation, that given two arguments licensed by a predicate, and in the absence of syntactic information, the first argument in a sentence is more likely than not to be interpreted as an actor rather than as an undergoer of a given action. However, rather than attributing this regularity to extra-linguistic knowledge, I follow the intuition that this systematicity in the way semantic roles are organized in syntactic representation follows from a syntactically relevant semantic representation that

(a) is independent from syntax and (b) does not go away even after more complex grammatical principles develop. Moreover, given that this organization is independent from syntactic representation, I assume that it can emerge as a system of correspondence whenever syntactic principles of linking fail to be properly implemented (or as I will propose below, fail to be implemented 'on time').

One piece of evidence for a semantically based linking rule of this sort comes from research on pidgin languages. Interestingly, pidgins seem to show consistent preservation of canonical order of arguments (agent/experiencer first) that is independent of the word order of languages involved in the pidginization process (Bickerton, 1981). This has been attributed to the fact that, in the presence of conflicting grammatical principles from the different languages involved (in other words, syntax is unreliable), speakers of the different languages unconsciously choose the syntactic linking that best resembles semantic linking (taken to be invariant across languages) for the purposes of establishing reliable communication.

Along similar lines, Klein and Perdue (1998) report on a longitudinal study on second-language learners (acquiring the language in a natural setting) where they find what they call 'the Basic Variety' (BV). This term refers to a type of language that emerges as the second language of adult learners (acquiring the second language in a natural setting) which may resemble the learners' target language – the language that the learners are attempting to acquire – but which has predictable grammatical features that are independent of the first language of the learner. The BV is characterized by lack of inflectional morphology, minimum number of closed-class items, and a very restricted number of syntactic configurations. Moreover, this language is organized according to a specific set of constraints (phrasal, semantic and pragmatic) that, again are independent of the native language of the learner. It is argued, as a result, that these organizational constraints of the BV reflect, in fact, the core attributes of the human language capacity (i.e. semantic system).

In this language, semantic constraints are argued to be concerned mostly with the semantic properties of arguments (or thematic roles) and the way they determine argument distribution in the sentence. One proposed generalization is that assignment of arguments to grammatical functions relies primarily on a principle of 'control asymmetry' [i.e. 'the noun phrase (NP)-referent with highest control comes first' (1998: 2)] between referents of nominals, such that an argument gets ranked higher or lower depending upon the amount of control that its referents exert. So, a verb like *break* <agent, theme> will show one assignment [*agent* – first, *theme* — second] respectively, given how different the *agent* is in terms of control from the *theme*. This contrasts with a verb, say, like *meet* which has very low controller asymmetry between the two licensed thematic roles.

This generalization, in addition to the pidgin evidence further supports the notion sponsored here that once syntactic principles of correspondence are made unavailable to the system – due to a processing impairment (Broca's aphasia), inability to acquire it (SLA), or availability of multiple systems (pidginization) – semantic principles, and, in particular, semantically based correspondence principles, are allowed to surface.

One additional piece of evidence for the existence of a syntax-independent organization of thematic roles comes from the work on syntax–semantics correspondence. Without entering into details, proposals on this issue operate on the generalization observed cross-linguistically, that, given two arguments licensed by a predicate, the one showing more agentive-like features (e.g. volition, causation, animacy, sentience and so forth) will have greater prominence in syntactic representation over less agentive arguments (i.e. it will occupy subject position). Proposals seeking to capture this kind of cross-linguistic regularity invariably invoke the notion of a lexico-semantic level of representation (e.g. argument structure), relevant for syntax but independent from syntactic structure, where thematic roles are organized according to semantic principles for the purposes of correspondence. This idea underlies generalizations such as the Thematic Hierarchy (e.g. Jackendoff, 1972, 1990b; Bresnan and Kanerva, 1989), and can also be found, for example, in Grimshaw's theory of argument structure (Grimshaw, 1990), Dowty's theory of Proto-Roles (Dowty, 1991), Baker's Uniformity of Thematic Assignment Hypothesis (UTAH) (1988) and Stowell's notion of 'Theta-grid'. Building on this insight I propose that *semantic linking* is in fact argument structure that in the absence of other information can potentially dictate the connections between arguments and syntactic functions.

Now, continuing with our system, assume also that in the intact brain, the system of correspondence is constrained in such a way that *syntactic linking* always prevails over *semantic linking* (I will call the constraint that keeps *semantic linking* from interfering the *linking* constraint). And suppose further that in the Broca's system the *linking* constraint is impaired. The consequence of this would be that even though both syntactic representation and argument structure are intact, the system now has, instead of one, two active linking mechanisms that, as a result, must *compete* against each other. This, in turn, means that whenever the two linking mechanisms agree, absence of the *linking* constraint is not apparent. However, whenever the two linking mechanisms yield conflicting correspondences (i.e. whenever semantic roles are reversed in syntactic representation) impaired comprehension, in the form of *chance* performance, will arise. I call the hypothesis that the constraint between these two mechanisms is not present in agrammatic comprehension associated with Broca's aphasia the Argument Linking Hypothesis (ALH).

As presented, however, this proposal begs the question of how it is possible that, in the presence of an intact syntactic system, *semantic linking* can emerge. In other words, what would the nature of the *linking* constraint be such that an otherwise suppressed mechanism can be allowed to operate and thus compete with *syntactic* linking? I propose here that the *linking* constraint is in fact a temporal constraint whose main effect is to keep a temporal differential in the unfolding of syntactic and semantic representations as comprehension progresses. As a result, syntactic mechanisms (including *syntactic linking*) will take place *before* any semantically based mechanism. However, if, for some reason, this temporal constraint is rendered inoperative, the two kinds of linking (*semantic* and *syntactic*) are left free to compete with each other.

Evidence for a 'slowed-down' lexical processor as a possible source of Broca's aphasia comprehension deficit has been well documented. Building on this, there are accounts proposing that even though Broca's patients are not unable to activate lexical meanings, for these patients, lexical activation in the form of priming seems to be 'temporally protracted', that is, it seems to have a 'slower-than-normal' time course (Prather, Shapiro, Zurif and Swinney, 1991; Zurif, Swinney, Prather, Solomon and Bushell, 1993 among others). I propose here that it is the inability to implement a fast-acting syntactic representation that allows the product of a semantic mechanism (i.e. linking by linear position) to emerge, off-line, for the purposes of sentence comprehension, and, as a result, to compete with *syntactic linking*. Such competition is only visible when the products of the two linking mechanisms differ (i.e. when thematic roles are reversed in syntactic representation).

The ALH predicts *above-chance* performance in actives, subject relatives and clefts because in these constructions both linking mechanisms (*syntactic* and *semantic*) coincide. So, in the sentence *The boy kissed the girl*, *the boy* (agent) is both first position and subject position, and *the girl* (goal) is both second position and object:

kissed <*agent, goal*>
agent = > first position = subject = > NP$_{the\ boy}$
goal = > second position = object = > NP$_{the\ girl}$

The ALH predicts *chance* performance in passives, object relatives and clefts, because in these constructions, the semantic and syntactic systems give conflicting correspondences. For a passive such as *The girl was kissed by the boy*, for instance, *syntactic linking* yields:

kissed <*agent, goal*>
agent = oblique = > (*agent* = NP$_{the\ boy}$)
goal = subject = > (*goal* = NP$_{the\ girl}$)

but *semantic linking* yields:

> kissed <*agent, goal*>
> *agent* = first position (agent = NP$_{the\ girl}$)
> *goal* = second position (goal = NP$_{the\ boy}$)

Given that the *linking* constraint is not available to force the system to opt for *syntactic linking*, both possibilities are, therefore, equally likely; so competition between these two systems ensues. This, in turn, results in *chance* performance (i.e. sometimes *syntactic linking* prevails and sometimes *semantic linking* does).

For object relatives and clefts a similar situation arises. In the subordinate clause of the sentence, *The girl that the boy kissed is tall*, *syntactic linking* yields:

> kissed <*agent, goal*>
> *agent* = > subject = > NP$_{the\ boy}$
> *goal* = > complementizer = > COMP$_{that}$[3]

but *semantic linking* gives:

> kissed <*agent, goal*>
> *agent* = first position (this results in *agent* = COMP)
> *goal* = second position (this results in *goal* = NP$_{the\ boy}$)

And again, it is the conflict between these two competing mechanisms that would yield *chance* performance.

So, as we see the ALH offers a view of Broca's agrammatic comprehension that does not capitalize on the presence of syntactic displacement, but that, instead, characterizes the comprehension as a slowing in the formation of the syntactic representation which, in turn, allows the product of the semantic system (semantically based correspondence between arguments and grammatical functions) to emerge.

Empirical evidence

One way to investigate which of these two hypotheses has correctly characterized the pattern of impairment observed is by teasing apart syntactic displacement and reversal of semantic roles. This, in turn, can be done by testing a construction that accommodates syntactic movement analogous to that observed in constructions for which performance is impaired – a construction that involves movement out of object position – but which does not cause deviation from the canonical order of thematic roles. Furthermore, in light of the formulation of the TDH, it is necessary that such a construction does not provide for the possibility of compensating mechanisms such as an 'agent first' strategy which could 'mask' the deficit. Such a case is afforded by unaccusativity or split intransitivity.

In what follows, I present a summary of the main issues regarding unaccusativity and a discussion of some empirical work that investigates how it plays out in Broca's agrammatic comprehension. To forecast, the results of that work will reveal, supporting the ALH, that once canonical order of semantic roles is controlled, Broca's comprehension performance does not necessarily show impairment in the presence of object movement. This type of evidence thus points to the system of correspondence as a likely locus of the deficit.

Unaccusativity

The Unaccusative Hypothesis, attributed to the work of Paul Postal and David Perlmutter [see Pullum (1991) for an interesting account of the history of this proposal] captures the observation that intransitive verbs divide into two subgroups based on their syntactic behaviour and that such difference in behaviour is correlated with semantic properties of the arguments they select. Intransitives that select semantic arguments with agentive-like properties are called unergatives (e.g. run, jump, sleep...) and intransitives that select arguments that exhibit undergoer-like characteristics are called unaccusatives (e.g. arrive, fall, bounce...).

In English, one important syntactic contrast attributed to unaccusativity involves the resultative construction. A fact about the resultative phrase in the resultative construction is that it can only be a predicate of the direct object of the verb as in the sentence *The girl watered the tulip flat* (the tulip became flat, not the girl) never of a subject or oblique complement (Simpson, 1983). Now, consider the following contrast:

1   a.* Carmen ran tired
     b. The river froze solid

(1a) is ungrammatical under the interpretation that 'Carmen' (*agent*) became tired as a result of running. (1b) on the other hand, is grammatical under the interpretation that 'the river' (*theme/undergoer*) solidified as a result of becoming frozen. So, even though neither 'ran' nor 'froze' license a syntactic object, only (1a) is ungrammatical under the resultative interpretation. This observation is taken to suggest that even though in (1b) 'the river' is in subject position, it is behaving like a direct object at some level of representation.

This type of evidence thus argues for the proposal that, in contrast to arguments of unergatives, arguments of unaccusatives are actually displaced constituents that, in underlying representation, are base-generated in object position.[5] The two distinct syntactic representations are thus illustrated as follows:

2   a. unergative [NP [V]] underlying representation
                    [NP [V]] surface representation
     b. unaccusative [e [V NP]] underlying representation
                    [NP$_i$ [V t$_i$]] surface representation

Finally, one additional difference between unergatives and unaccusatives is that only unaccusatives allow causative alternates (i.e. a transitive counterpart of the unaccusative) where the subject of the unaccusative has semantic properties analogous to those of the object of the causative. So, for some unaccusative verbs such as *shatter*, *brake* or *spin* there is a transitive (causative) version that differs from the intransitive one in that it licenses, in addition to an underlying object, an underlying subject: *The mirror shattered* (intransitive) vs. *John shattered the mirror* (causative transitive). I will refer to this type of unaccusative verb as *alternating unaccusative*.

In sum, unaccusative verbs (both alternating such as *shatter* and non-alternating such as *arrive*) are monadic (one argument) verbs that initially link their argument to the underlying *object* position. (This argument then moves to subject position in surface representation leaving behind an argument trace.) Unergatives, on the other hand, are also monadic predicates that, in contrast, link their argument directly to the underlying *subject* position.

Granting that the Unaccusative Hypothesis has correctly captured the contrast just described, we have then a testing ground for our two hypotheses. This is so because unaccusativity allows us to distinguish syntactic movement from thematic role ordering. As we can see in Table 5.1, the construction with the unaccusative (a) provides us with the possibility of a contrast that eliminates the confound of thematic role reversal (there is only one licensed thematic role), and replicates, for all relevant purposes, syntactic movement (i.e. object movement) of the kind observed in passives (b) and object relatives (c):

Table 5.1. Different constructions — same displacement

Constructions	Thematic structure licensed by the verb
a. *The vase*$_i$ broke t$_i$	*<theme>*
b. *The vase*$_i$ was broken t$_i$ by the boy	*<agent, theme>*
b. *The vase*$_i$ that$_i$ the boy broke t$_i$ is green	*<agent, theme>*

Having presented the linguistic phenomena that constitutes the basis for our conditions, I will now discuss the experimental evidence that seeks to distinguish between the two competing proposals (TDH and ALH).

Syntactic displacement in Broca's comprehension

In a recent study (Piñango, 1998), I investigated the comprehension performance of four subjects: two Broca's patients (RD and JC) classified as Broca's based on the BDAE (Goodglass and Kaplan, 1972) and two neurologically intact control subjects. Both agrammatic Broca's aphasic patients were medically stable and at least two years post-onset. Equally important, both patients exhibited the prototypical cluster of Broca's symptoms such as effortful, telegraphic and poorly articulated speech, and restricted vocabulary. Lesioned areas for both Broca's patients included the anterior inferior LH (area roughly associated with Broca's area). And, most importantly, their lesions excluded Wernicke's area.

These two patients also showed the sentence comprehension pattern associated with Broca's aphasia, revealed in *above chance* performance in so-called adjectival 'passives' (containing neither thematic reversal nor object movement), and *chance* performance in verbal passives. So, the profile these patients exhibit ensured that they were truly representative of the Broca's aphasia population.

All four subjects were tested in sentential constructions with unergatives, alternating unaccusatives and non-alternating unaccusatives using the sentence–picture matching task.[5] Table 5.2 shows an example of each experimental sentence per condition.

Table 5.2. Experimental conditions

Condition	Sample sentence
Unergative	The girl clapped because of the boy
Unaccusative non-alt.	The girl$_i$ fell t$_i$ because of the boy
Unaccusative alt.	The girl$_i$ spun t$_i$ because of the boy

Again, notice that all three sentence types contain monadic predicates. To make these sentences similar to the thematic configuration of the passive and object relative and cleft, a second argument was introduced in an adverbial phrase (i.e. *because*-phrase). In contrast to the passive and object relative/cleft, however, this argument has no syntactic or semantic connection (regarding selectional restrictions) with the main verb of the sentence. So, as we can see, sentences for the three conditions differ syntactically *only* with respect to whether the argument is base-generated in pre- or post-verbal position.

The next point to be addressed concerns the predictions that both the TDH and the ALH afford us. For alternating unaccusatives the TDH yields two different predictions depending on our assumptions regarding the participation of the thematic role in the adverbial-phrase. If we assume that the Broca's patient will analyse the thematic role of *causer* as a simple variant of *agent*, then the prediction is *chance*. This is so because as the strategy incorrectly assigns agency to the subject NP (which is left dangling after the object trace has deleted), it leaves the sentence with one *agent* and a *causer*:

> *The girl$_i$* spun t$_i$ because of *the boy* – intact representation
> *theme*   *causer*

> *The girl* spun * because of *the boy* – agrammatic representation
>   ?   *causer*

> *The girl* spun * because of *the boy* – strategy applies
> (agent/causer)   *causer*

If on the other hand, we assume that *agent* and *causer* are *not* equivalent for the purpose of Broca's comprehension (as they are not equivalent in the normal language system), then the prediction would be *below-chance* (i.e. systematic reversal). There are two main reasons for this: (1) alternating unaccusatives do license *agents* in their alternative causative form (e.g. *The girl spun the boy*) and (2) the pictures in the test offer a possible *agent* (in both pictures one of the characters is performing an *agent*-like action). From this it follows that, in the agrammatic representation, the NP bearing the role of *agent* will be systematically selected over the NP bearing the role of *causer* (which, given its adverbial function, is not even required to be present in the picture for the purposes of the semantic well-formedness of the sentence). This results in *below-chance* performance.

For non-alternating unaccusatives (e.g. *arrive, fall, stumble...*), the TDH's prediction is again modulated by our assumptions regarding the thematic role of the adverbial. The prediction for non-alternating unaccusatives is *chance* if we assume competition between *agent* and *causer*. By contrast, the prediction is *below-chance* if no competition is assumed. This is so because once the strategy has applied, the subject NP is marked as *agent* and although Broca's patients know that unaccusatives do not license *agents*, an *agent* is provided in the pictures. This makes it possible for the patient to ignore the sentence and just focus on the information the pictures provide, to make her or his response.

Finally, assuming that subjects are base-generated in their surface representation position, for unergatives, the TDH predicts that Broca's performance should be *above-chance*.

By contrast, the ALH predicts that Broca's patients will perform *above-chance* across the three conditions. This prediction arises from the fact that in all three conditions there is only one argument per predicate which by both *syntactic linking* and *semantic linking* should correspond to the subject position (= first position). Table 5.3 summarizes the predictions.

Table 5.3. Summary of predictions

Constructions	TDH		ALH
	Assuming competition between *agent* and *causer*	Not assuming competition between *agent* and *causer*	
Unergative	Above-chance	Above-chance	Above-chance
Unaccusative (alt)	Chance	Below-chance	Above-chance
Unaccusative (non-alt)	Chance	Below-chance	Above-chance

The results for our two Broca's patients were calculated individually using binomial tests performed on proportion correct for each condition. These tests revealed that both patients, just like the two neurologically intact subjects, performed *above-chance* across all three conditions (JC performed 93% correct on unergatives and non-alternating unaccusatives, and 100% correct on alternating unaccusatives; RD performed 86.6% correct on unergatives, 93.3% correct on non-alternating unaccusatives and 80% correct on alternating unaccusatives).

Let us consider these results for a moment. As we can see, each proportion correct falls well within the range of performance also observed, in most Broca's patients, for constructions such as the active and subject relative. And, just like performance in actives and subject relatives, each proportion correct for unaccusatives contrasts with performance observed for the syntactically analogous passive and object relative.

This point is relevant here because, as we may recall, our two Broca's patients were shown to exhibit the classical pattern of performance just described; thus corroborating that they were representatives of the Broca's agrammatic population. It is these two sets of results combined – good performance in actives/subject relatives contrasting with impaired performance in passives/object clefts and relatives, on one hand, and good performance on unaccusatives on the other – that allow us to put our findings in perspective.

This new perspective is, in fact, the observation that whatever causes impaired comprehension for passives and object relatives, is not present in the sentences with unaccusatives. Given the experimental controls implemented in the study, it seems that this factor is reversal in the canonical order of thematic roles in syntactic representation and not argument movement.

Summary and conclusions

The observation that first motivated this work was that even though the locus of the Broca's agrammatic deficit was syntactic in nature – and in particular, the result of argument-chain disruption – impaired comprehension (i.e. *chance* performance) could only be observed *when syntactic movement brought about reversal of thematic roles*. This is what gave rise to the ALH.

If the results reported here tell us anything about Broca's agrammatic comprehension, they tell us that if thematic-role reversal is prevented, syntactic movement does not account for the deficit. This is made clear in cases such as the present because the possibility of a compensating mechanism like the *agent*-first strategy – that could mask the underlying deficit – is not available. This finding, together with the other contrasts discussed, thus force us to re-evaluate movement-based accounts in general and, in particular, the TDH given that, as formulated, it cannot account for the evidence.

By contrast, and as the ALH suggests, this evidence opens the door to enquiry regarding representational and processing mechanisms involved in the connection between argument structure and syntactic functions. This new perspective still circumscribes the deficit to syntax, but places it at the interface between these two types of representation.

The evidence presented here furthers our understanding of the basis of Broca's agrammatic comprehension by discriminating between two different processes – syntax-lexico-semantics correspondence vs. syntactic displacement. Given the lesion localizing value of this syndrome, this evidence further allows us to posit that it is the timely correspondence between syntactic and semantic representation via syntactic mechanisms that seems to depend on the integrity of Broca's area.

Acknowledgements

Research for this work was supported by NIH grants DC 02984 and DC 00081. I owe a great deal to Edgar Zurif, Nalama Friedmann and Ray Jackendoff for very helpful comments and advice in the preparation of the manuscript.

Notes

[1] Traces in theta positions are created whenever syntactic movement of a noun phrase (NP) takes place from its base-generated position in underlying representation to its final landing site in surface representation.

In Government and Binding theory (Chomsky, 1981), argument traces are the recipients of thematic information which is assigned structurally by the verb to its arguments. The connection between the object position (where the trace is) and the subject position (where the antecedent has moved to) is established by a so-called argument chain that links the antecedent with its *trace*. The following illustrates the process:

(2) e is chased *the bird* by the cat (underlying representation)

(3) *The bird*$_i$ is chased t$_i$ by the cat (surface representation)
     |___chain ___| Move-alpha

[2.] This notion is, of course, not new. It can be found in different guises in Caramazza and Zurif (1976), Linebarger, Schwartz and Saffran (1983), Caplan and Futter (1986) and Hagiwara and Caplan (1990) among others. However, those proposals differ from the present instantiation of that insight, in that they consistently attribute sensitivity to canonical order to a *heuristic*, and in doing so, fail to see the import that such regularity has for the linguistic system. That is, they fail to see that rather than being just a reflection of extra-linguistic knowledge, sensitivity to canonical order of thematic roles by Broca's aphasic patients could be a reflection of a preserved *linguistic* principle.

[3.] The complementizer is analysed as the bearer of the thematic role assigned by the verb in the subordinate clause. It is connected via predication to the subject of the matrix clause *the girl*. The subject NP of the matrix clause is assigned a thematic role by the verb phrase of the matrix clause *is tall* .

[4.] I have presented the Unaccusative Hypothesis only to the extent that it serves the experimental conditions required here. Nevertheless, the scope and implications of this proposal goes well beyond what I have discussed. See Zaenen and Maling (1984), Grimshaw (1987) and Levin and Rappaport-Hovav (1995) among others for in-depth discussion of this proposal and its implications.

[5.] For each sentence there were two pictures depicting the correct and semantically reversed interpretation of the sentence.

Chapter 6
Levels of linguistic representation in Broca's aphasia: Implicitness and referentiality of arguments

JENNIFER E. BALOGH AND YOSEF GRODZINSKY

Introduction

This study investigated agrammatic representation of two properties – one semantic and one phonetic, and the way these interact with the patients' comprehension abilities of passive constructions. We investigated two elements which we varied systematically: (1) referential properties of moved noun phrases (NPs) in subject positions, and (2) implicit (i.e. phonetically realized) and overt *by*-phrases in passive. We obtained results indicating that both elements significantly affect performance, yet in different ways. We also tested Wernicke's aphasics, to see whether damage in different brain regions would yield different results in this type of test.

Background

The Trace Deletion Hypothesis (TDH, Grodzinsky, 1986, 1990) was designed to handle the agrammatic deficit in receptive language (comprehension, grammaticality judgment, and real-time processing, cf. Grodzinsky, in press, for review). Specifically, the deficit to syntactically moved elements is at its centre. Yet the complexity of the ever-increasing body of data has changed the standard pattern of loss and sparing, and given certain novel theoretical considerations, a reformulation was forced. The result is a more restrictive, precise theory – the Trace-Based Account (TBA, Grodzinsky, 1995a). We examined two aspects of language to see which of them, if any, influences comprehension patterns typically observed in agentive passives. The properties of interest here are *referentiality* and *implicitness* of arguments. They were chosen for a reason – referentiality is a semantic property of NPs, whereas implicitness regards phonetic realization. We wanted to investigate the interaction between processes involving different levels of linguistic representation subsequent to brain damage. Specifically, we wanted to see how a purely syntactic deficit interacts with a semantic and a phonetic level. We thus varied our stimuli systematically along semantic and phonetic dimensions, seeking to chart out the interaction between these properties, and the movement-related properties of the passive construction.

A semantic property – referential vs. non-referential arguments

As experiments become more sophisticated, charting ever more precisely the intricate performance patterns revealed in aphasia, it is becoming increasingly clear that referential properties of at least some arguments play an important role in the comprehension deficit in agrammatic aphasia. The first relevant finding is due to Hickok and Avrutin (1994) who tested agrammatic comprehension on four types of questions, along two dimensions: questions pertaining to subject (1a,c) vs. object (1b,d) position, and those expressed by *which* (1a,b) vs. *who* (1c,d). The findings they obtained are in parentheses:

1   a. Which boy pushed the girl?[1]   (above chance)
      b. Which boy did the girl push *t*?   (chance)
      c. Who pushed the girl?   (above chance)
      d. Who did the girl push *t*?   (above chance)

Previous experiments have documented subject/object asymmetries in constructions with movement – subject extractions yield normal performance, whereas object extractions are performed at chance (cf. Grodzinsky, 1990 for a review). Yet here there was a surprise: on the structure in (1d), namely on the *who* object question, the patients were, unexpectedly, above chance, in apparent violation of the TDH.

    Why would such an asymmetry be observed? There are differences between the two types of questions, motivating this experiment in the first place: first, *which*-questions (but not *who*-questions) are 'Discourse(D)-linked', requiring reference to previous discourse (cf. Pesetsky, 1987). The question in (1a), for instance, presupposes the existence of a set of boys, already been mentioned in the discourse, from which one boy will be picked. It is pragmatically odd (although syntactically well formed) to ask questions (1a and b) if there are no boys around. Thus, the interpretation of *which*-questions requires both syntactic and contextual information. By contrast, no such requirements exist for *who*-questions. Questions (1c and d) can be asked without presupposition, and the answer does not pick an element from a previously established set. Their interpretation is based only on intrasentential (syntactic and lexical) information.

    Second, certain intricate tests on multiple questions reveal fine differences between the two: Superiority (Chomsky, 1973) can be violated by *which*-questions under certain conditions, but not by *who*-questions. The Superiority Condition requires that, in multiple questions, a moved *wh*-element cannot cross another:

2   a.   *Who$_i$* did you persuade t_i to read *what*?
     b.   ??*What$_i$* did you persuade *who(m)* to read t_i?

These cases constitute part of a generalized Superiority Condition – Rizzi's (1990) Relativized Minimality (RM). Specifically, Rizzi proposes that a moved element can never cross a like element, a proposal which accounts for a variety of syntactic phenomena across movement types (cf. Grodzinsky and Finkel, 1998 for a study of RM in aphasia). Yet, as Pesetsky (1987) observes, Superiority can be violated under certain circumstances, for instance, where *which*-questions are involved, (3) is the *which* analogue of (2), yet the contrast observed in the latter disappears [compare (2b) to (3b)]:

3   a.   *Which man$_i$* did you persuade t_i to read *which book*?
     b.   *Which book$_i$* did you persuade *which man* to read t_i?

This difference, noted by Pesetsky, had led Cinque (1990) to propose a refinement to Rizzi's RM, and argue in favour of the existence of two types of movement relations, or chains: Binding (1a and b) chains, and Government chains [covering (1c and d) in the present context] where only the former are D-linked. This distinction helps Hickok and Avrutin to claim that in agrammatism only the Binding chain is disrupted, which presumably explains the asymmetry in the agrammatic data. Left unexplained, though, is the normal performance of the agrammatics in (1a). Moreover, this claim does not generalize to the problem agrammatics have in passive (cf. Grodzinsky, 1995a for a critique of this claim).

Let us consider the matter in some more detail. Following his observations, Pesetsky (1987) attempts to exploit the distinction between D(iscourse)-linked and non-D(iscourse)-linked questions, as well as the Superiority-related syntactic differences between the two question types, to propose the following:

4   a.   Non-D-linked phrases are quantifiers and adjoin to S$^|$
     b.   D-linked *wh*-phrases are not quantifiers.

This conclusion means that non-D-linked phrases (*who*) are not referential (because quantifiers never are), whereas D-linked phrases (*which* NP) are referential.

Pesetsky's ideas have been used by a reformulated account of agrammatism, the TBA (Grodzinsky, 1995a). Following the distinction between D-linked and non-D-linked moved phrases, the TBA claims that cognitive strategies (and specifically, the default strategy of the TDH) apply to referential elements only,[2] leading to a reformulation of the default strategy used in agrammatism. Specifically, quantifier-like, non-referential *wh*-expressions are outside the scope of the strategy and therefore, non-referential NPs are exempt from it:

5 *R(eferential) strategy* (Grodzinsky, 1993b)
Assign a referential NP a role by its linear position if it has no Theta-role.

The interaction between the TBA and the R strategy gives precisely the desired results. (1a and b) are accounted for as before. In (1b) the strategy-assigned role on the NP [which boy] conflicts with that assigned to the subject NP [the girl], yielding chance performance. (1a) is a subject question, thus if there is movement, then it is correctly compensated for by the R strategy. But now consider (1c and d). Because *who* is a non-referential expression, it is exempt from the R strategy. Thus in both cases, no role is assigned strategically to the *wh*-word. As a result, only one role is assigned [to the subject in (1c) and to the object in (1d)], and, given the intactness of lexical knowledge in agrammatism, the correct semantic role of the thematically dangling NP can be easily inferred.[3] Hence above-chance performance is predicted, fitting the data – old and new – precisely.[4]

This claim can be generalized in the following way: in movement-derived structures, with agentive predicates, one would expect chance performance if the moved constituent is extracted from object position, and is referential (6a). Yet, when the antecedent of the trace is non-referential (6b), performance should go up to normal levels, even though it contains an agentive predicate and a trace in object position, as we saw in (1d). This is so because the strategy (whose interaction with the rest of the thematic representation brought about guessing) is now absent, and hence the patient can infer the correct thematic representation from the available information.

6 a. The man is pushed *t* by the boy
   b. Every man is pushed *t* by a boy

Although counterintuitive, this prediction has received some initial empirical support from a preliminary study by Saddy (1995), who found a difference in the performance of a Broca's patient on regular passive sentences (6a), and passives in which the subject is a quantified expression (6b). Specifically, performance in the latter was better, even though it is ostensibly more 'complex'. We decided to try and obtain this finding for a group of aphasics in a broader experiment, and we thus presented the test materials in conjunction with the other structures we intended to test.

It is important to emphasize that, because the passive construction is not fully understood in linguistics (cf., for instance, Jaeggli, 1986; Baker, Johnson and Roberts, 1989; Grimshaw, 1990; Pesetsky, 1994; Fox and Grodzinsky, 1998), and as many details of its analysis remain highly controversial, the debate on agrammatism should not take it as the centre-piece of the deficit (indeed, it has not, at least as far as the TBA has been concerned). Results involving the passive are valuable only if (a) they are taken in conjunction with other structures (as has been the case with the TBA), or (b) they are used to obtain contrastive results, through interaction with other (grammatical or non-grammatical) factors. This latter approach has been taken in the present study. Specifically, we used the passive as part of an effort to discover what information remains intact in the agrammatic's syntactic representation.

A phonetic property – implicit vs. overt arguments

A related question that focuses on the representation of arguments and their corresponding ϑ-roles involves short passives, namely, what happens when there is no *by*-phrase? For a short passive in which the *by*-phrase is truncated, such as 'the man is hit', the only argument present is the derived subject. For agrammatics, this argument will have no thematic label because it has been moved and has left a trace behind which is ultimately deleted. The prediction the TBA has crucially depends on the type of theory it is coupled with regarding the representation of the deleted *by*-phrase, in particular, the status of implicit arguments. The issue, in brief, revolves around the syntactic function and representation of the missing *by*-phrase. A hallmark of linguistic theory is the requirement that a predicate cannot appear at any syntactic level of representation with more or less arguments than those listed in the lexicon for that predicate. The short passive is a clear counterexample of this requirement, as it manifests with and without the external argument of its predicate:

7   a. John is hit by Bill
     b. John is hit

One way of getting around this dilemma is to argue that the missing argument is syntactically active and represented, even though it is silent and invisible (i.e. implicit). To see how it works, consider first an independent proposal aimed at solving other problems posed by the passive. This proposal states that the ϑ-role of the external argument is 'absorbed' in the passive morphology during the process of passivization (e.g. Jaeggli, 1986, and many others). The *by*-phrase, if present, on this account, receives its ϑ-role from the passive morphology through some process (whose precise nature is highly controversial, cf. Jaeggli, 1986; Baker et al., 1989; Grimshaw, 1990; Fox and Grodzinsky, 1998). If the *by*-phrase is deleted, as in short passive, that ϑ-role remains in the passive morphology, and, importantly, it is syntactically active, as can be seen in the following contrasts (cf. Manzini, 1983):[5]

8   a.   The captain sank the ship to collect insurance money
     b.   The ship was sunk by the captain to collect insurance money
     c.   The ship was sunk to collect insurance money
     d.   *The ship sank to collect insurance money

The question is, what is the subject of the infinitival purpose clause *to collect insurance money* (or, in technical terms, what controls the PRO subject of the infinitive). Clearly, in (8a) it is *the captain*. Similarly in (8b) it is *the captain* again, controlling the PRO from inside the *by*-phrase, perhaps. Yet in (8c) we discover, surprisingly, that the meaning of the sentence remains unchanged, namely, that there is someone out there who sank the ship to collect insurance money, even though this someone is not represented by an overt NP. This gives us an indication that there is some argument, implicitly represented, which functions as the subject of the infinitive. Importantly, this argument must be present in the active construction, as seen from (8d). In this example, the verb *sink* has one less argument for reasons that are lexical, not syntactic. In this structure, nothing can control the PRO and hence the sentence is ungrammatical. The conclusion is that there is an implicitly represented argument in the short passive. When coupled with the idea that the external ϑ-role is absorbed in the passive morphology, one possible solution to the dilemma regarding short passives is that the implicit argument is represented in the passive morphology.

Returning now to agrammatic aphasia, we are left with an open question: does the implicit argument in the short passive interact with the default strategy and affect performance? There are several possibilities to consider. (1) The implicit argument does not manifest itself in the patient's representation, and does not interact with the strategically assigned agent θ-role. In this case, the patient would perform below chance because the only ϑ-role they would have in their representation is agent, assigned to the subject NP (which should be theme according to normal grammar); because there is no other ϑ-role around to compete with the subject for agency, the agrammatic would assume that the subject is the one performing the action and would reverse the correct interpretation systematically. (2) The implicit argument is represented, and is pitted against the strategically assigned agent in the subject position of the short passive. If this is the case, then comprehension would be at the same level as the agentive passives, because the argument in the *by*-phrase – whether overt or implicit – would appear in the thematic representation. On this account, the subjects would be guessing because they have two agents, even though there is only one overt argument. Chance performance will thus help us make a case for the existence of a phonetically unrealized, implicit agent. (3) Finally, the patients could perform above chance, a result which would indicate a 'fill-in-the-blank' strategy. On this (remotely possible) account, there is no implicit ϑ-role, and no strategy as the one assumed by the TBA. The patient uses the information available, namely that there is one ϑ-role which needs to be assigned to one NP. Because there is only one option, the patient makes the correct choice.

All these considerations led us to test short passives in conjunction with the other experimental conditions we constructed.

Methods

Subjects

Twelve subjects participated in the study: four neurologically intact control subjects, four agrammatic Broca's aphasic patients and four Wernicke's aphasic patients.

All normal control subjects were right-handed, native speakers of English, who had never experienced any head injury and whose eyesight and hearing were corrected to normal. Ages ranged from 69 to 72 with an average education of 13.5 years.

All agrammatic Broca's aphasic patients were medically stable, with at least two years since the date of stroke. All were right-handed native speakers of English whose eyesight and hearing were corrected to normal. The ages ranged from 59 to 79 with an average education of 13.5 years (see Table 6.1).

All Wernicke's aphasic patients were medically stable, with at least five years post onset. All were right-handed, native speakers of English whose eyesight and hearing were corrected to normal. The ages ranged from 59 to 71 with an average education of 11.25 years (see Table 6.2).

Materials

Stimulus items consisted of 20 token sentences for each of the four different sentence types: actives, agentive passives, short passives and quantified passives. A verb appearing in an active structure, such as 'pay', was also represented in an agentive passive, short passive and quantified passive. The following is an example of each sentence type:

1. The man pays the woman.   (active)
2. The man is paid by the woman.   (agentive passive)
3. The man is paid.   (short passive)
4. Every man is paid by the woman. (quantified passive)

Table 6.1. Lesion sites and speech impairments for the four agrammatic Broca's aphasic patients in the study

Patient	Onset	Lesion site	Speech
FA	1992	CT Scan 1992 Left CVA – CT scan is unremarkable	Non-fluent Paraphasias Agrammatic Telegraphic Verbal and oral apraxia
FC	1973	MRI 24/10/94 Very large left dorsolateral frontal lobe lesion involving almost all of the inferior and middle frontal gyri. Lesion includes all of Broca's area and the white matter deep to Broca's area. The lesion continues superiorly and includes the lower two-thirds of the pre-motor, motor and sensory cortex and the white matter and periventricular white matter deep to these areas. There is no lesion in the temporal and parietal lobules	Non-fluent Dyspraxia Agrammatism
RD	1976 and 1977	CT Scan 1978 Two left frontal lesions – Broca's area with deep extension across to left frontal horn – lower motor cortex (face and lips) left temporal lobe sparing more than one-half of Wernicke's area	Non-fluent Telegraphic
WF	1994	CT Scan 21/5/94 A large lateral frontal lesion, a large lesion in the frontal opercullum, and two small lesions, one in the motor cortex and the other in the caudate putamen anterior limb of the internal capsule	Non-fluent Agrammatic Impaired articulation Long latencies in speech

CVA: cerebro-vascular accident.

Eighty short stories were created, one for each sentence, in order to create an appropriate discourse context, against which the truth-value judgment task can be properly performed.[6] Each story involved several visual aids, including figurines which represented the characters, and in some cases an additional prop that pertained to the context of the story such as a canoe or currency. See Appendix 6.1 for instructions and example stimuli.

Design

A truth-value judgment task (Crain and McKee, 1985) was used to assess patients' comprehension of the sentences. This experimental design ensured that an appropriate licensing context for the scenario depicted in the sentence was created for the subject, thus avoiding any computational overload involved in generating a discourse context.

Table 6.2. Lesion sites and speech impairments for the four agrammatic Wernicke's and anomic aphasic patients in the study

Patient	Onset	Lesion site	Speech
CC	1984	CT Scan 17/7/84 Left hemisphere lesion involving portion of posterior temporal lobe with superior extension into supramarginal and angular gyrus areas (surface and deep) and large occipital lobe lesion	Fluent Anomic
WD	1991	CT Scan Left hemisphere lesion in the posterior part of the inferior section of MCA; one-quarter of Wernicke's area deep to supramarginal gyrus	Fluent Anomic
NL	1987	CT Scan 13/10/95 Decreased density in the left posterior parietal area. Although it is adjacent to the posterior body of the left lateral ventricle, it does not appear to distort the ventricle. Low attenuation region in the left posterior temporo-parietal region	Fluent Naming difficulty Paraphasias Neologisms
JM	1986	CT Scan 22/1/86 Vague patchy lesion involving the temporal isthmus and the posterior/superior portion of putamen and insular area. Patchy, superior lesion extension in the posterior supramarginal and angular gyrus areas with deep extension across to the border of the body of the left lateral ventricle-interrupting pathways of the arcuate fasciculus	Fluent Anomic Paraphasic

Half of the sentences required a 'yes' response and half required a 'no' response, with rotations among the verbs for each sentence type so that each agentive verb was in two 'yes' and two 'no' contexts, making all items counterbalanced.

All stories involved two figurines except for those which were followed by quantified passive sentences. These stories used six characters instead of two so that one type of character (e.g. one of the three dog figurines) could perform an action on each of the three characters of the other type (e.g. on each of the three pig figurines). We included three of each type of character so that the subject could not use the number of characters (one vs. three) as part of a strategy to deduce which character type was fulfilling a certain θ-role in the sentence.

Sentences and their respective stories were presented in a random order.

Procedure

The experiment was conducted in four sessions, with a break during each session, so that only 15 sentences and stories were presented at a given time. This was done to avoid overtaxing the patients.

Patients were given explicit instructions about what would take place during the session and what they were expected to do. An example was presented so that subjects could observe a demonstration of what they would be asked to do. Then subjects were given a short practice session in which they responded as they would during the actual experiment, but feedback was given and reasons for correct responses were explained.

First, each of the figurines for a given story was identified to the patient and given a name, for example, 'This is the girl'. This was done to establish a discourse context for the characters who later appeared in the sentences. Then the subject heard a short story while the experimenter acted out the scenario using the figurines. After the story, a sentence was read, and the subject was to decide whether the sentence matched or did not match the story.

To circumvent severe speech-production impediments, the patient was asked to respond by pointing to a picture. The patient made a 'yes' response by pointing to a coloured smiling face with the word 'yes' printed underneath or a 'no' response by pointing to a frowning face with the word 'no'.

To ensure that the patient understood the story and sentences to the fullest, each sentence was repeated twice. The patients were also encouraged to ask the experimenter to have either the sentence or story or both be repeated as many times as the patient wished.

After the patient made a response by pointing, the response and number of repeats were recorded.

Results

Neurologically intact elderly control data

The data for the control subjects were broken down into sentence type and compared to chance using a two-tailed t-test. For each sentence construction, $n = 20$ with a hypothesized mean of 10 ($p = 0.50$) when at chance, given that in all cases there was a binary choice. Table 6.3 presents the p-value for each condition:

All sentence types are significantly above chance. A pairwise comparison of means showed that there were no significant effects for any sentence types and that there was no significant difference between overall 'yes' vs. 'no' responses.

Table 6.3. Elderly control data (each sentence type compared to chance performance)

Sentence type	Mean	p-value
ABOVE CHANCE		
Active	18.75	<0.0001
Agentive passive	18.75	0.0004
Short passive	19.25	0.0003
Quantifier passive	19.75	<0.0001

Aphasic patient data

Broca's aphasics

The data for the Broca's aphasics were broken down into sentence type and compared to chance using a two-tailed t-test. For each sentence construction, $n = 20$ with a hypothesized mean of 10 ($p = 0.50$) when at chance. Table 6.4 presents the p-value for each condition:

Table 6.4. Broca's aphasic data (each sentence type compared to change performance)

Sentence type	Mean	p-value
ABOVE CHANCE		
Active	17.75	0.0125
Quantifier passive	17.00	0.0046
AT CHANCE		
Agentive passive	14.50	0.0979
Short passive	14.50	0.1970

Actives and quantifier passives are significantly above chance, whereas performance on agentive passives and short passives is at chance.

Pairwise comparisons of means showed that there was a significant effect for actives vs. agentive passives [$F(1,15) = 4.768, p = 0.0453$, MSe = 4.431], actives vs. short passives [$F(1,15) = 4.768, p = 0.0453$, MSe = 4.431] (see Table 6.5).

Table 6.5. Pairwise comparison of means for Broca's aphasics

	Active	Passive	Short	Quantified
Active		+	+	
Passive	+			
Short	+			
Quantified				

+ Represents a significant difference between conditions.

Wernicke's aphasics

The data for the Wernicke's aphasics were also broken down into sentence type and compared to chance using a two-tailed t-test. For each sentence construction, $n = 20$ with a hypothesized mean of 10 when at chance. Table 6.6 presents the p-value for each condition for these patients.

Table 6.6. Wernicke's aphasic data (each sentence type compared to change performance)

Sentence type	Mean	p-value
ABOVE CHANCE		
Active	19.25	<0.0001
Quantifier passive	17.50	0.0109
AT CHANCE		
Agentive passive	13.75	0.0650
Short passive	14.25	0.2238

Actives and quantifier passives are significantly above chance, whereas performance on agentive passives and short passives is at chance.

A pairwise comparison of means (see Table 6.7) showed that there was a significant effect for actives vs. agentive passives [$F(1,15) = 9.233$, $p = 0.0083$, MSe = 6.553], actives vs. short passives [$F(1,15) = 7.630$, $p = 0.0145$, MSe = 6.553].

Table 6.7. Pairwise comparison of means for Wernicke's aphasics

	Active	Passive	Short	Quantified
Active		+	+	
Passive	+			
Short	+			
Quantified				

A comparison of the performances of the two clinical groups using an ANOVA revealed no significant effects across the groups for any given condition.

A comparison of 'yes' and 'no' responses revealed that, for Broca's aphasic patients, there was no significant difference between the responses for each condition, and therefore showed no overall response bias in either direction. A comparison of Wernicke's aphasic patients did not present any significant difference between 'yes' and 'no' responses for any sentence type. There was also no significant effect for 'yes' and 'no' responses across the two clinical groups.

An item analysis revealed no clustering of errors. An analysis of word frequency (Francis and Kucera, 1982) for the verbs in this sentence type revealed that there is no correlation between word frequency and errors.

Discussion

Summary of results

Of the complex array of findings in Tables 6.5 and 6.7, here are what we consider to be the two types of main results of this experiment:

A. Differential performance of agrammatic (and Wernicke's) aphasics:
    1. Agentive passives with quantified (i.e. non-referential) subjects are above chance.
    2. Short, truncated passives are comprehended at chance, and significantly different from their agentive active counterparts.
B. No group differences.

A complex performance array

Referentiality

With regard to referentiality, our results replicate Saddy's (1995) experiment — that is, the patients' comprehension of the passive construction improves when the moved constituent includes a non-referential quantifier. This finding lends further support to the R strategy.

Implicit arguments

Next when considering the role of implicit arguments on comprehension patterns, we see that the absence of an argument does not improve comprehension for passives with transitive verbs. As with the passive construction, patients performed at chance on the short passives. This result leads us to the conclusion that a second ϑ-role, even if not realized at Phonetic Form, is represented in the syntax, and is part of the thematic representation. A conflict with the strategically assigned agent ϑ-role on subject thus arises, forcing the patient to resort to guessing. A conclusion along these lines strongly suggests that the patients have access to information about covert arguments in their representation and that the ϑ-roles mapped on to covert arguments play a crucial role in a patient's interpretation.

Group differences (or lack thereof)

We found no difference between the groups. We expected such differences, but failed to find them. Opponents of clinical groupings in aphasia might take this result as a decisive argument against clinical groupings in aphasia. This conclusion is clearly unwarranted. There is no reason to expect no overlap in the comprehension performances of agrammatic Broca's and Wernicke's aphasics. The deficits the two groups suffer need not be, and in fact could hardly be imagined to be, completely distinct. There is, as yet, little understanding of the underlying deficit in Wernicke's aphasia, but the known differences among these two patient types (most prominently in speech production, but also in many receptive tasks as well) suffice to establish the validity of the clinical groupings. Only adherence to the traditional clinical schema, and further experimentation, will reveal the true picture. Indeed, as experiments on receptive abilities in aphasia are becoming more and more subtle, a syntactic disturbance of some sort is gradually being revealed in Wernicke's aphasia (cf. Grodzinsky and Finkel, 1998 for another study documenting a systematic syntactic deficit in this syndrome). The currently available experimental results present a very mixed picture, still quite difficult to understand. The array of findings does include a host of receptive tasks on which Wernicke's aphasics are quite different from Broca's aphasics (cf. for instance, Shapiro, Gordon, Hack and Killackey, 1993; Zurif, Swinney, Prather, Wingfield and Brownell, 1995). Thus, although certain involvement of temporo-parietal areas in syntactic processing is beginning to emerge, it is not very likely to be a consequence of the same disruption evidenced in agrammatism.

Acknowledgements

The preparation of this manuscript was supported by NIDCD grant CD-00081 to the Aphasia Research Center, Boston University School of Medicine, and Israel-U.S. Bi-national Science Foundation Grant 97-00451 to Tel Aviv University.

Appendix 6.1: Instructions for passive study

This experiment may seem silly at first because it uses children's toys. The reason we use toys is so that you can see action while listening to a story. We don't mean to be insulting and apologize if it seems offensive to you.

For this experiment you are going to hear a series of 30 short stories. The characters in each story will be introduced to you before you hear the story. While you are listening to the story, you will see the characters acting out what is happening.

After each story you will hear a sentence that will either match or not match the story. Here's an example:

This is a boy. This is an elephant.

Practice Story 1
The elephant doesn't like little boys. When the elephant sees the boy, he runs away. The boy chases after the elephant until they both run out of breath.

Practice Sentence 1
The boy chases the elephant. (repeat)

Does the sentence match what happened in the story? If you think it did, point to the smiling face. Now don't worry about whether the story could actually happen in real life. For many of the stories you will have to stretch your imagination. All we want you to do is to determine whether the sentence after the story matches or doesn't match what happened in the story. Here's another sentence:

Practice Sentence 2
The elephant chases the boy. (repeat)

Does this sentence match what happened in the story? (wait for response) Right, the boy was the one who was doing the chasing, not the elephant. Because this sentence doesn't match the story, you would point to the frowning face.

· Listen carefully to each story and the sentence that follows so that you can decide whether the sentence matches the story. Be sure to look at the characters while each story is being read.

This isn't a timed test, so you can take as long as you want to decide whether a sentence matches or doesn't match the story. You can have the sentence repeated as many time as you want. You may also ask that the entire story be repeated.

Make sure that you pay attention to who is doing what in the sentence. Decide on each sentence very carefully. If you think that the sentence matches what happened in the story, point to the smiling face. If you think that the sentences DOES NOT match what happened in the story, point to the frowning face.

Do you have any questions? Here are some more practice stories.

EXAMPLE STIMULUS ITEMS

Active
The characters are an Indian and a swimmer
The story is   *The Indian is having a coughing fit. The swimmer wants to help, so he hits the Indian on the back to help stop the coughing.*
The sentence is   *The Indian hits the swimmer.* (repeat)
(Correct response is **NO**)

Agentive Passive
The characters are a muscle man and a boy
The story is   *The muscle man is living in the boy's closet and pays rent every month. When the first of the month arrives, the muscle man gives the boy some money.*

The sentence is   *The muscle man is paid by the boy.* (repeat)
(Correct response is **NO**)

Quantified Passive
The characters are three men and three mice
The story is   *The mouse has just won some money from playing*
    bingo. The mouse wants to pay off some of his debts.
    He gives some money to the first man, then the
    second man and finally to the third man.
The sentence is   *Every mouse is paid by the man.* (repeat)
(Correct response is **NO**)

Short Passive
The characters are a robot and a horse
The story is   *The horse has been painted for a special festival.*
    Now the horse wants to wash the paint off, but he
    can't reach some of the spots. The robot takes a
    sponge and helps the horse get clean.
The sentence is   *The robot is washed.* (repeat)
(Correct response is **NO**)

Notes

[1.] Traces in subject position were not annotated here, because their presence or absence from the representation has no empirical consequences in the present cases. Cf. Grodzinsky (1990: 170).

[2.] Referentiality is used here in the manner common in linguistics, namely, in a sense that does not require reference in the world, but rather, in the universe of discourse. An element is thus used referentially when it refers to a member of a set that has been pre-established in discourse. Cf. Chomsky (1981), Pesetsky (1987), Rizzi (1990), Cinque (1990).

[3.] As Na'ama Friedmann correctly points out, an additional assumption is necessary here: the language-processing device must be capable of carrying out this inference in a way that has access to all the data structures that are required, namely the syntax as well as the argument structure. This is a non-trivial, yet a rather plausible assumption.

[4.] One issue still needs to be addressed. When a non-referential NP is left without a θ-role, the strategy is not applied and agrammatics must infer which θ-role the moved constituent receives in these cases. But why shouldn't they be able to make the same inference for all other passive constructions? The answer is that there is an order among the steps applied to a representation. The agrammatic interpretive system first identifies an argument without a θ-role and uses the default strategy to assign one to that constituent. If the NP is non-referential, the strategy is withheld. Only after this step has taken place can the agrammatic begin extracting meaning from the syntactic structure. It is at this point that the patient chooses which agent bears the correct theta-role for agentive passives, or if need be, makes an inference regarding the correct θ-role to a moved non-referential constituent.

[5.] See also Jackendoff 1972 for other arguments to the same effect, e.g. *the price was decreased willingly* vs. **the price decreased willingly*.

[6.] With one exception (Hickok and Avrutin, 1996), no study of agrammatic comprehension has ever had an appropriate discourse context. This point should not be overlooked by critics of results of experiments on agrammatic comprehension.

Chapter 7
Verb-finding problems in Broca's aphasics: The influence of transitivity

ROEL JONKERS

Introduction

Studies on the retrieval of lexical verbs in Broca's aphasics are often restricted to the comparison of the scores on action and object naming in these patients. It has been reported that, for Broca's aphasics, verbs were more problematic than nouns, whereas, for anomics, nouns were more problematic than verbs (e.g. Miceli, Silveri, Villa and Caramazza, 1984). Basso, Razzano, Faglioni and Zanobio (1990), however, found no differences between action naming and object naming for the Broca's and anomic aphasics they tested. Finally, Williams and Canter (1987) and Kohn, Lorch and Pearson (1989) found a specific deficit for verbs as compared to nouns in all aphasics, who participated in their studies, among which there were Broca's aphasics and anomics.

Bastiaanse (1991) showed, in an experimental study, that the performance of aphasics in action naming may depend on the type of the elicited verb. The results of her study showed that name-relation of a verb with a noun influenced the scores of Dutch Broca's and anomic aphasics on an action naming task.

It has been suggested that several factors might influence noun retrieval (e.g. word frequency, imageability, familiarity), but it is unclear which factors influence the retrieval of verbs. From the study of Bastiaanse it can be concluded that *name-relation with a noun* is one of these factors. As Broca's aphasics suffer from a syntactic deficit, it might be assumed that a syntactic factor plays a role in verb retrieval in these patients. Therefore, in the present study, the effect of such a factor on verb retrieval, i.e. *transitivity*, will be evaluated.

Lexical entries of a verb contain, next to its meaning and its phonological form, several kinds of syntactic and semantic information. The different syntactic and semantic elements of the lexical entry will be outlined below, following Chomsky's Government and Binding (Chomsky,

1981) and Principles and Parameters (1986) framework. The lexical entry
of *to give*, for example, consists of the following information:

1   *give*   * syntactic category: V
             * syntactic complements (subcategorization): [_NP NP] or
                [_NP PP]
             * argument structure: (x,y,z)
             * thematic structure: (agent, theme, recipient)

The lexical entry contains word-class information. In this case, the
syntactic category V (verb) is indicated. The syntactic complements represent the subcategorization frame of the verb. The subcategorization frame
specifies the syntactic environment into which a verb can be placed. The
verb *to give* has two possible complement structures. One [_NP NP] (NP,
noun phrase) is necessary in order to produce sentences like (2).

2   The boy gives the girl (NP) the book (NP)

In this case, apart from the subject, an indirect object and a direct object
are produced. Instead of the production of an indirect object, an oblique
complement may be produced by using a prepositional phrase (PP). This
accounts for sentences like (3).

3   The boy gives the book (NP) to the girl (PP)

Subcategorization is used as well-formedness information. Sentences
must satisfy the *Projection Principle* (Chomsky, 1981):

4   Projection Principle: representations at each syntactic level are
     projected from the lexicon, in that they observe the subcategorization
     properties of lexical items

This means that sentences must satisfy the complement structure of a
verb. Therefore, a sentence like (5) is ungrammatical because one complement is missing.

5   *The boy gives the girl

The argument structure representation is also used as syntactic well-
formedness information. The verb *to give* has three arguments which are
represented as variables (x, y, z). Argument structure is concerned with the
number of participants expressed by the conceptual representation. The
verb *to give* requires three participants, a *giver*, a *receiver* and a *given
object*, as is represented in (6).

6   [The boy x] [gives [the girl y] [the book z]]

The arguments that fall within the domain of the verb (y, z) are *internal arguments*, whereas (x), falling outside this domain, is an *external argument*.

Verbs requiring three arguments are called three-place verbs. Apart from these, one-place (e.g. *to skate*), two-place (e.g. *to grind*), and four-place verbs (e.g. *to exchange*) exist. All arguments must be specified in a sentence in order to make it well-formed, following the Projection Principle. The example in (5) is not well-formed because one complement/argument position is unspecified.

The argument structure of a verb interacts with the specification of its semantic or thematic roles, the thematic structure. The verb *to give* has three thematic roles, *the agent* (the one who performs the action of giving), *the theme* (the thing that is given) and *the recipient* (the one who gets the thing that has been given). During sentence construction, thematic roles are assigned to the arguments of the verb. Within the Government and Binding framework, this assignment is based on the *Theta Theory*. This theory states that Theta-roles are assigned to arguments by a Theta-assigner (i.e. lexical categories like verbs, prepositions, nouns and adjectives). This assignment is constrained by the *Projection Principle* [see (4)] and the *Theta Criterion* (Chomsky 1981):

7   Theta Criterion: each argument bears one and only one Theta-role, and each Theta-role is assigned to one and only one argument

This means that the thematic roles, specified by the lemma, will be assigned to the arguments in a one-to-one fashion. The verb *give* will assign the role of agent to *the boy*, the one who performs the action, the role of theme to *the book*, the object that is given and the role of recipient to *the girl*, the person who is receiving the theme, as is shown in (8).

8   GIVE (boy$_{agent}$, book$_{theme}$, girl$_{recipient}$)

In order to create the syntactic structure, the complements have to be mapped on to the structure in (8). The NP *boy* will be subject, the NP *book* will be the direct object, and the NP *girl* will be the indirect object.

Thompson, Lange, Schneider and Shapiro (1997) showed that the *verb argument structure* influenced verb retrieval of Broca's aphasics in test conditions. No effect of argument structure was found in a confrontation verb-naming task, but sentence production was influenced by the number of arguments a verb requires: Broca's aphasics preferred the least complex verbs, namely verbs requiring one argument, like *to ski*. Comparable scores were found by Kiss (this book) in a sentence construction task in two Hungarian Broca's aphasics. Thompson, Lange, Schneider and Shapiro (1997) also reported that the number of possible argument structure arrangements played a role. Two-place verbs, in which both arguments are obligatory, have only one argument structure. This is the case for *to kiss*, as is clear from examples (9) and (10).

9   The man kisses the woman
10 *The man kisses

These verbs are called *obligatory two-place verbs*. There are, however, also verbs in which one of the arguments is not obligatorily realized, the so-called *optional two-place verbs*. For these verbs the absence of the internal argument does not make the sentence ungrammatical as is shown in examples (11) and (12).

11 The man drinks a beer
12 The man drinks

These *optional two-place verbs* are supposed to have two argument structure arrangements, one with and one without the internal argument realized in the syntax.

Thompson and colleagues found that sentences with verbs with only one argument structure were more often correctly produced than sentences with verbs with more possible argument structures.

Thompson, Lange, Schneider and Shapiro (1997) also showed that the *thematic structure* of the verb plays a role in sentence construction. They found the following order of difficulty: sentences with only an Agent or an Experiencer role were significantly more often correct than sentences with a Theme/Patient role, which in turn were better preserved than sentences with a Goal/Location role.

The studies of Thompson and colleagues and Kiss (this book) focused on the *argument structure* and the *thematic structure* of the verb. The present study concentrates on the *subcategorization frame* of the verb by considering the effect of the syntactic factor *transitivity*.

As far as is known, the effect of transitivity on verb retrieval has never been studied in aphasia research. The influence of this factor on verb retrieval in children has been investigated by Davidoff and Masterson (1996). They showed that children have more problems in naming pictures of intransitive than of transitive verbs, suggesting that intransitive verbs are more difficult to retrieve than transitive verbs.

In the present study, verb retrieval, in isolation and in sentence context, by Broca's aphasics will be investigated, focusing on the effect of *transitivity*.

Methods and materials

Subjects

The study included 15 Broca's aphasics, all native speakers of Dutch. The diagnosis of Broca's aphasia was based on the classification of the Dutch version of the Aachen Aphasia test (Graetz, De Bleser and Willmes, 1992) and was confirmed by clinical judgment of a person who did not know the patients. Patient data are presented in Table 7.1.

Table 7.1. Patient data for the Broca's aphasics

	Age	Aetiology	Localization	MPO	Sex	Paresis
B1	45	CVA-L	Parieto-temporal (CT)	77	m	+
B2	78	CVA-L	Subiuscular/internal capsules (CT)	29	f	+
B3	38	CVA-L	Area middle cerebral artery (CT)	154	f	?*
B4	54	CVA-L	Basal fronto-temporal (CT)	4	m	+
B5	61	CVA-L	Area middle cerebral artery	11	m	+
B6	72	CVA-L	Fronto-temporal (EEG)	89	m	+
B7	65	CVA-L	Parietal (CT)	5	m	+
B8	53	CVA-L	Occipito-parietal (CT; slight signs)	12	m	rec.
B9	66	CVA-L	Area middle cerebral artery (CT; large area)	7	m	+
B10	51	CVA-L	Area middle cerebral artery (EEG: fronto-temporal)	10	f	+
B11	63	CVA-L	Fronto-temporal (CT)	125	f	+
B12	47	CVA-L	Temporo-parietal (CT)	38	m	+
B13	48	CVA-L	Area middle cerebral artery (CT; large area)	5	f	rec.
B14	62	CVA-L	Area middle cerebral artery (CT)	56	m	rec.
B15	71	CVA-R	No information available	9	m	+
Mean:	58.3			46.7		

Notes: CVA: cerebro-vascular accident; L: left hemisphere; R: right hemisphere; CT: CT scan; EEG: electroencephalography; MPO: months post onset; m: male; f: female; rec.: recovered; *: congenital missing right arm.

All Broca's aphasics suffered from a single stroke. The patients did not have major auditory or visual problems.

For comparison the scores of a group of 15 healthy subjects were used who matched the aphasic group in age, sex and social background.

Materials

A confrontation naming (action naming) and sentence production (sentence construction) task were administered. Because naming-to-picture tests were used, all items were highly imageable. Both tests consisted of 60 items. The verbs in the action naming and in the sentence construction task were different, but the items in action naming matched fully with the items of the sentence construction test.

The verbs were controlled for *transitivity* (see below) and two other linguistic factors: instrumentality of the verb and name relation to nouns (cf. Bastiaanse, 1991).

Frequency

The items in the tests were matched for word-frequency using the CELEX frequency lists for Dutch (Burnage, 1990).

Transitivity

To evaluate the effect of transitivity, the 60 verbs were divided into two subgroups: 30 intransitive verbs and 30 transitive verbs. *Transitive verbs* were those verbs that required a direct object, like *to grind* and *to scratch*, whereas *intransitive verbs* were verbs that could not have a direct object, like *to fence* and *to swim*. The transitive verbs were matched for frequency with the intransitive verbs.

Within the class of transitive verbs, some grammarians make the distinction between pure transitives and so-called *pseudo-transitives*. Pseudo-transitives are, in principle, transitive but these verbs may also occur without a direct object, like *to milk* or *to saw*. Nevertheless, these verbs are considered to be transitive. Thompson, Shapiro, Tait, Jacobs and Schneider (1996) indicate that with these verbs one always assumes an object, although it is not always lexicalized (e.g. in order to milk there always has to be some animal that is milked, like a cow).

The verbs that were used in the subtests were not specifically controlled for the thematic structure of the verb. All items, however, concerned action verbs, which means that the thematic structure was either *Verb + agent, theme/patient* (transitive verbs), or *Verb + agent* (intransitive verbs).

An example of each type of verb with respect to transitivity, taken from the verb tests, is presented in Figure 7.1.

Reliability

Reliability of the tests was calculated using the odd–even coefficients. Correlation between the two parallel halves was corrected for length using the *Spearman–Brown formula*. The odd–even reliability for *action naming* was $r = 0.96$ ($p < 0.001$) and for *sentence construction* was $r = 0.90$ ($p < 0.001$).

Procedure

All aphasics were tested using the same procedure. A picture was shown to the patients and they were asked to tell either in one word (*action*

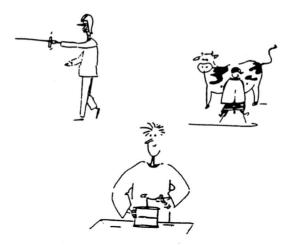

Figure 7.1. Examples of an intransitive verb (*fencing*; Dutch: *schermen*), a pseudo-transitive verb (*milking*; Dutch *melken*) and a transitive verb (*grinding*; Dutch: *malen*).

naming) or in a sentence (*sentence construction*) what the person on the picture was doing. Both tests started with two examples. Patients who gave an inadequate response to one of these were corrected. If patients produced (part of) a sentence for the examples of action naming they were asked to react in one word. In cases where patients produced an incomplete sentence in sentence construction they were requested to produce a complete sentence. After the examples no more feedback was given. There was no time limit; self corrections were allowed and scoring was based on the final answer.

The tests were administered in two sessions. Action naming was carried out in one session and sentence construction in another. The order of the two sessions was assigned randomly to the patients such that some of the patients were tested first with the sentence construction test and others with the action naming test. There was at least a four-day interval between the sessions.

Scoring

The test sessions were tape-recorded. In scoring action naming, a count was given if the correct verb was retrieved. It was not considered whether it was produced as a single word. This means that if a patient produced the correct verb within a (part of a) sentence, then the reaction was counted as correct. In sentence construction, a count was first given in terms of whether the intended verb was retrieved. Next, the production of subjects and objects in sentence construction was examined. This was done in order to account for a possible relation between an effect of transitivity and the realization of the syntactic complements that belong to the verb.

Overall results on verb retrieval

Overall results for action naming and sentence construction by both groups are presented in Table 7.2.

Table 7.2. Mean and standard deviation (*sd*) of action naming and sentence construction scores

	Action naming	Sentence construction
Broca's aphasics (*n* = 15)		
Mean (*sd*)	22.6 (*10.8*)	24.1 (*9.6*)
Controls (*n* = 15)		
Mean (*sd*)	54.6 (*2.9*)	53.4 (*3.3*)

The controls performed significantly better than the Broca's aphasics in verb retrieval in isolation [t(28) = 11.1, $p < 0.001$] and in sentence context [t(28) = 11.2, $p < 0.001$]. Verb retrieval in isolation did not differ from verb retrieval in sentence context within both subject groups [*Broca's aphasics*: t(14) = 0.80, $p > 0.05$; *controls*: t(14) = 1.19, $p > 0.05$].

The effect of transitivity on verb retrieval

Table 7.3 shows the results for the action naming and sentence construction tasks of the Broca's aphasics and the controls with respect to effect of *transitivity* on verb retrieval.

Table 7.3. Mean and standard deviation (*sd*) of action naming and sentence construction scores with respect to the factor transitivity

	Action naming		Sentence construction	
	Transitive	Intransitive	Transitive	Intransitive
Broca's aphasics				
Mean (*sd*)	12.7 (*6.0*)	9.9 (*5.0*)	12.1 (*4.6*)	12.0 (*5.4*)
Controls				
Mean (*sd*)	27.5 (*1.6*)	27.1 (*1.8*)	27.3 (*1.7*)	26.1 (*2.3*)

Transitive verbs received higher scores than intransitive verbs by the Broca's aphasics at the word level [t(14) = 4.70, $p < 0.001$]. At the sentence level, this difference disappeared [t(14) = 0.09, $p > 0.05$]. No effect of *transitivity* was found in the controls [*action naming*: t(14) = 0.69, $p > 0.05$; *sentence construction* t(14) = 2.09, $p > 0.05$].

In conclusion, transitivity was shown to have an effect on verb retrieval in isolation, but not in sentence context, by the Broca's aphasics. It was decided that a closer look at the data of the Broca's aphasics was needed in order to find out why an effect of transitivity was found only at the word level and not at the sentence level.

A closer look at the data

The individual scores on action naming and sentence construction showed that within the group of Broca's aphasics, different performance patterns could be distinguished. Half of the patients performed better in action naming than in sentence construction, whereas the other half showed the opposite pattern. The patients were divided into two subgroups on the basis of this distinction in their scores on the two tests. The patients in subgroup 1 (7 subjects) performed better in action naming than in sentence construction, whereas those in subgroup 2 (8 subjects) had a better performance in sentence construction than in action naming. In Table 7.4, the mean group scores are presented.

Table 7.4. Mean and standard deviation (*sd*) of action naming and sentence construction scores in the subgroups

	Action naming	Sentence construction	Statistics
Subgroup 1 ($n = 7$) Mean (*sd*)	25.6 (*11.7*)	20.6 (*10.9*)	$p < 0.02$
Subgroup 2 ($n = 8$) Mean (*sd*)	20.0 (*10.0*)	27.1 (*7.6*)	$p < 0.002$
All Broca's aphasics Mean (*sd*)	22.6 (*10.8*)	24.1 (*9.6*)	$p > 0.05$

The scores in Table 7.4 reveal that, although the group of Broca's aphasics as a whole had comparable scores for action naming and sentence construction, subgroup 1 was significantly better in verb retrieval at the word level than at the sentence level [$t(6) = 3.62$, $p < 0.02$], whereas for subgroup 2 the opposite was true [$t(7) = 6.00$, $p < 0.002$].

Transitivity had an effect on action naming but not on sentence construction when the scores of all Broca's aphasics were looked at. Below, it will be considered whether the same holds for the subgroups.

First, a descriptive analysis will be presented. In Figure 7.2, the individual scores on verb retrieval in isolation and in sentence context by the Broca's aphasics are depicted in two scatterplots. In these scatterplots a division into subgroups is projected in relation to transitivity.

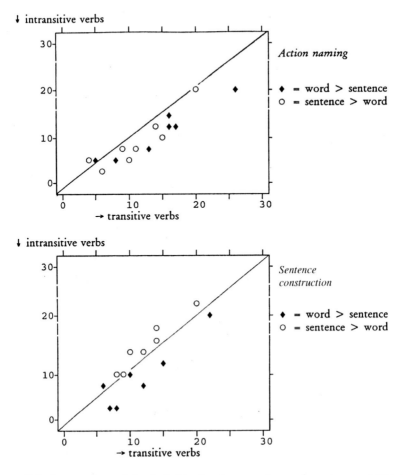

Figure 7.2. Scatterplots of the individual action naming and sentence construction data with respect to the factor *transitivity*. Subjects with higher scores in verb retrieval in isolation are represented by a diamond, subjects with higher scores in verb retrieval in sentence context are represented by a circle.

The sloping line in the scatterplots in Figure 7.2 divides the group into those patients who were better in retrieving transitive verbs than intransitive verbs (depicted under the line) and those who showed the opposite pattern (depicted above the line). Twelve of the 15 patients had higher scores for transitive than for intransitive verbs in action naming. This shows that the effect of transitivity, found at the word level, is present in most of the individual patients. This contrasts to the pattern found for verb retrieval in sentence context. The scores of all except two patients in subgroup 1 are plotted below the sloping line, meaning that they performed better on transitive verbs than intransitive verbs. All patients in subgroup 2 showed the opposite pattern: a better performance on intransitive than transitive verbs.

The effect of transitivity will be discussed further in the following section.

The effect of transitivity on the scores of the subgroups

Table 7.5 gives the scores of both subgroups on action naming and sentence construction with respect to transitivity. In Figure 7.3, these scores are depicted graphically.

Table 7.5. Mean and standard deviation (*sd*) of action naming and sentence construction scores in the subgroups with respect to *transitivity* (subgroup 1: action naming > sentence construction; subgroup 2: sentence construction > action naming)

(a) Verb retrieval in isolation

	Transitive	Intransitive	Statistics
Subgroup 1 (*n* = 7) Mean (*sd*)	14.4 (*6.8*)	11.1 (*5.0*)	$p < 0.02$
Subgroup 2 (*n* = 8) Mean (*sd*)	11.1 (*5.1*)	8.9 (*5.1*)	$p < 0.05$

(b) Verb retrieval in sentence context

	Transitive	Intransitive	Statistics
Subgroup 1 (*n* = 7) Mean (*sd*)	11.4 (*5.6*)	9.1 (*5.6*)	$p < 0.05$
Subgroup 2 (*n* = 8) Mean (*sd*)	12.6 (*3.8*)	14.5 (*3.9*)	$p < 0.01$

Subgroup 1 (action naming > sentence construction) was significantly better in naming transitive than intransitive verbs in isolation [$t(6) = 3.58, p < 0.02$] and in sentence context [$t(6) = 2.49, p < 0.05$]. Subgroup 2 (sentence construction > action naming) also produced significantly more transitive verbs than intransitive verbs in isolation [$t(7) = 3.00, p < 0.05$], but, at the sentence level, this group was significantly better in retrieving intransitive than transitive verbs [$t(7) = 3.91, p < 0.01$].

From these results it can be concluded that, although the Broca's aphasics behave like a homogeneous group at the word level, they split into two subgroups at the sentence level, behaving differently with respect to the effect of *transitivity*.

The production of subjects and objects

The production of subjects and objects was evaluated in order to find out whether *transitivity* played a role in the production of these verb comple-

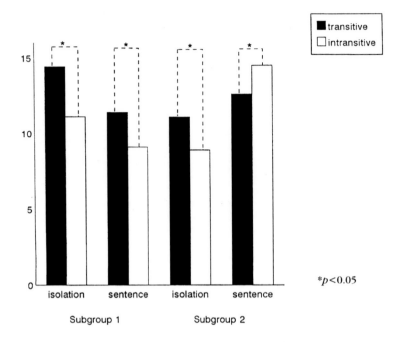

Figure 7.3. The subgroups' performance on the factor *transitivity* at the word and the sentence level (subgroup 1: action naming > sentence construction; subgroup 2: sentence construction > action naming).

ments. Subject and object complements were only counted in sentences containing the target verb. Table 7.6 gives an overview of the results of the subgroups with respect to the subject and object production and the effect of *transitivity*.

Subject complements were produced significantly more often with a transitive than with an intransitive verb in subgroup 1 [t(6) = 2.55, $p < 0.05$]. No difference was found between intransitive and transitive verbs as far as the number of subject complements is concerned in subgroup 2 [t(7) = 0.73, $p > 0.05$].

An object was produced with 64% of the transitive verbs in subgroup 1, whereas subgroup 2 only produced an object with 28% of the transitive verbs. It was, however, not always necessary to produce an object. If only obligatory contexts for objects were taken into account, the number of objects reached 80% for subgroup 1 and 38% for subgroup 2. Subgroup 1 produced both the subject and the object with 55% and subgroup 2 with 16% of the transitive verbs.

It is clear that at the sentence level the two groups of Broca's aphasics not only differed with regard to the effect of *transitivity* on verb retrieval, but also in the production of subjects and objects.

Table 7.6. Mean and standard deviation (*sd*) of the proportional scores for the production of subjects and objects in the subgroups (subgroup 1: action naming > sentence construction; subgroup 2: sentence construction > action naming)

(a) Production of subjects

	Transitive	Intransitive	Statistics
Subgroup 1 ($n = 7$)			
Mean (*sd*)	80.6 (*17.6*)	57.9 (*36.4*)	$p < 0.05$
Subgroup 2 ($n = 8$)			
Mean (*sd*)	61.7 (*33.4*)	55.2 (*29.3*)	$p > 0.05$

(b) Production of objects

	Object	Subject + object
Subgroup 1 ($n = 7$)		
Mean (*sd*)	63.9 (*22.2*)	55.4 (*22.1*)
Subgroup 2 ($n = 8$)		
Mean (*sd*)	27.8 (*17.3*)	15.7 (*15.6*)

Summary

Verb retrieval in Broca's aphasics and the effect of the syntactic factor *transitivity* on retrieval was analysed. No differences were found between the scores for action naming and sentence construction. *Transitivity* was shown to affect verb retrieval. When simple actions had to be named, transitive verbs were better preserved than intransitive verbs. The test for sentence construction revealed that two groups could be distinguished. The first group was better in action naming than in sentence construction, but the effect of *transitivity* was the same in verb retrieval in isolation and sentence context: transitive verbs were better preserved than intransitive verbs. Subject complements were more frequently produced with transitive than with intransitive verbs. The number of object complements realized with the transitive verbs was relatively high.

The second group demonstrated an opposite effect of *transitivity* at the word and sentence levels. Contrary to verb retrieval in isolation, this group retrieved more intransitive than transitive verbs in sentence context. The number of subjects and objects obtained with the correctly retrieved verbs was relatively low.

Discussion

The present study showed that verb retrieval in Broca's aphasics may be influenced by the type of verb. A syntactic factor, transitivity, played a role in verb retrieval in these aphasics. Transitive verbs were easier to retrieve than intransitive verbs in action naming. In this final section, why transitive verbs were easier to retrieve for all Broca's aphasics at the word level and only for some of them at the sentence level will be discussed.

The effect of *transitivity* is explained by focusing on the syntactic information that is stored with the verb. First, however, whether the effect that was found could be due to the fact that the present study only used tests containing pictorial materials will be discussed. With respect to *transitivity*, Canseco-Gonzalez, Shapiro, Zurif and Baker (1990) have pointed out the possible influence of visual artifacts. According to these authors, there is a relationship between argument structures and visual information: 'argument structures are shaped by the form in which visual information is parsed' (p. 402). In a therapy study concerning comprehension in a Broca's aphasic, they found that an extra element depicted in the picture facilitated performance only when this element was an argument. When this element was an adjunct it disrupted learning. It may thus be argued that transitive verbs in the present study were easier to name because all arguments were depicted and that the intransitive verbs were more difficult, despite the fact that often an element that was not an argument was in the picture. The picture for the verb *to climb*, for example, showed a mountain. For verbs like *to kneel*, however, nothing but the agent was depicted.

This is a serious point to consider but there is reason to assume that the relation between the number of elements in the picture and the number of arguments was not the critical factor in the present study: the transitivity effect in half of the aphasics was different at the word and the sentence level. For these aphasics, in sentence context, intransitive verbs were easier to retrieve than transitive verbs, whereas facilitation of an argument arose at this level in the Canseco-Gonzalez et al. study.

Davidoff and Masterson (1996) considered that the children's problems with intransitive verbs may have been due to difficulties in picture interpretation. Therefore, they performed a second study using video clips. Comparable results were found, showing that the transitivity effect did not seem to be due to the interpretation of pictures.

As already stated, the performance of the Broca's aphasics will be explained by concentrating on the syntactic information that a verb carries. According to Thompson, Lange, Schneider and Shapiro (1997), all syntactic information is activated when the verb is retrieved, not only in sentence construction, but also in action naming. They argue that if the number of arguments and subsequently the amount of syntactic information increases, the verb becomes more difficult to activate. This implies that transitive verbs, bearing more syntactic information than intransitive verbs, would be more difficult to retrieve than intransitive verbs, both in isolation and in sentence context. However, this was not found in the present study: a larger amount of syntactic information does not make verbs more difficult to retrieve. On the contrary, transitive verbs were easier than intransitive verbs.

The amount of syntactic information stored with the verb was demonstrated to affect sentence construction. It will, however, be argued that the more syntactic information a verb contains, the more difficult sentence construction becomes, but not that the verb becomes more difficult to retrieve.

In the next subsection, the fact that transitive constructions are more frequent in language and thus they are easier to retrieve than intransitive verbs for patients with a syntactic deficit will be discussed.

The transitivity effect in action naming

The lexical entry of a transitive verb differs from the one of an intransitive verb, as is shown in Figure 7.4.

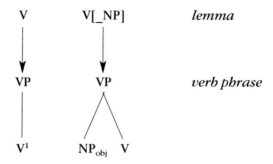

Figure 7.4. The lexical entry of an intransitive and a transitive verb.

The verb phrases that belong to these verbs also differ. For an intransitive verb only a V is specified, for a transitive verb both a V and an NP object is specified.

In the spontaneous speech of normal subjects, transitive verbs with one internal argument occur three times more often than intransitive verbs. This is true not only for Dutch but also for English and Hungarian (Bastiaanse, Edwards and Kiss, 1996; Edwards and Bastiaanse, 1997). A related study showed that in spontaneous speech, Broca's aphasics also used more transitive than intransitive verbs, just like normal subjects (Bastiaanse and Jonkers, 1998). The relative high frequency of transitive verbs is also demonstrated by the CELEX frequency list of Dutch (Burnage, 1990): from the 150 most frequent main verbs, 100 are transitive whereas 50 are intransitive.

Arguing along the lines that there is a direct relationship between activation threshold and frequency of use, transitive verbs in general are more often retrieved and as a consequence the corresponding verb phrases are more readily available. Broca's aphasics suffer from a syntactic impairment, making it difficult to process all the syntactic information that is stored with a verb. This also holds for verb retrieval in isolation, meaning that even for verb retrieval in isolation the verb phrases are retrieved. As the verb phrase for transitive verbs is more readily available, these verbs are easier to produce than intransitive verbs.

The ability of the Broca's aphasics to retrieve verbs is then assumed to be influenced by a syntactic factor: the frequency of a grammatical construction. Note that this has nothing to do with word frequency. The intransitive and transitive verbs were matched for word frequency.

The transitivity effect in sentence construction

The transitivity effect that was found at the word level for all Broca's aphasics was found at the sentence level in only those patients who scored higher in action naming than in sentence construction (subgroup 1). The patients who were better in verb retrieval at the sentence level (subgroup 2), produced more intransitive verbs than transitive verbs in sentence construction.

It is tempting to claim that those Broca's aphasics who were better in verb retrieval at the sentence level were less severely aphasic. If, however, the production of subject and object complements was taken into account, it was seen that subgroup 1 produced subjects relatively often, particularly when a transitive verb was activated. Also, in transitive sentences, the object was usually produced. This means that when these patients retrieved the verb, they tried to make complete sentences. Subgroup 2 produced fewer subject complements with both intransitive and transitive verbs and the patients in this group regularly omitted object complements, showing that they made 'incomplete sentences'.

Problems in sentence production are the core features of Broca's aphasia and therefore it is not surprising that both subgroups have problems in sentence production. The way these problems appear, however, differs.

Two patterns of sentence production problems

The fact that transitive verbs were easier to retrieve than intransitive verbs for subgroup 1 has already been explained with respect to action naming. In sentence construction, the patients in subgroup 1 tried to process all the syntactic information that is stored with a verb, in order to make a complete sentence. They often produced both the subject and an object complement. How does this explain the fact that they produced fewer verbs in sentence context than in isolation?

These patients wanted to process the complete amount of syntactic information that is stored with a verb in the lexicon, as is clear from the relatively preserved production of subjects and objects in those cases that the correct verb was retrieved. They were, however, often unable to process all the syntactic information, due to their syntactic problems. This led to problems in verb retrieval as such. In isolation, verbs were easier to retrieve, because at the word level, the syntactic information of a verb did not have to be processed in order to make a sentence.

The patients in subgroup 2 were better in verb retrieval in sentence context than in isolation. This suggests that they profited from a sentence frame in verb retrieval: a sentence frame fits with the syntactic information that is activated with the verb. Nevertheless, these patients did, of course, also have problems in sentence processing. They were unable to process the complete amount of syntactic information that was necessary for sentence construction, leading to, for example, the regular omission of object complements.

The preference for intransitive over transitive verbs in sentence context can be retraced to the fact that intransitive verbs contain less syntactic information than transitive verbs. Hence, the patients in subgroup 2 were able to construct a sentence frame, but they were unable to process a large amount of syntactic information in order to fill this sentence frame.

In sum, there are two ways in which the sentence production problems show up in the aphasics in the present study. Some patients tried to process all syntactic information in order to make complete sentences (i.e. with the subject and object complements), leading to verb production problems in sentence context. Other patients tried to produce simple sentences (i.e. without object complements), not using the complete amount of syntactic information, reducing the verb production problems in sentence context as compared to retrieval in isolation.

How do the results in this chapter relate to studies that considered the effect of verb argument and thematic structure on verb retrieval in Broca's aphasics?

Thompson, Lange, Schneider and Shapiro (1977) and Kiss (this book) found that Broca's aphasics preferred verbs with one argument in sentence production. This pattern fits with the pattern found for the subgroup in the present study that produced more intransitive than transitive verbs correctly. These patients also had a preference for simple sentences with only a subject and a verb.

The other subgroup produced more complex sentences. This differs from the outcomes of Thompson et al. and Kiss. The patients in this subgroup have, however, more problems with verb retrieval, as such, in sentence context than in isolation. Although Thompson and colleagues did not find such patients in their study, they concluded that it may be both the verb and its grammatical information that could lead to sentence production problems. According to them it is a 'complex mixture of verb and syntactic variables that influence sentence complexity and production' (Thompson, Lange, Schneider and Shapiro, 1997: 487).

Conclusion

From the results presented in this study, it may be concluded that the syntactic information stored with the verb plays an important role in verb retrieval for patients with a syntactic deficit. It was shown that more syntactic information does not make a verb more difficult to retrieve, but it does make sentence processing more difficult. In this respect, the results are in line with those of Thompson, Lange, Schneider and Shapiro (1997) and Kiss (this book), who found that in sentence construction Broca's aphasics preferred simple sentences with only one argument.

In the present study, patients reacted differently to the large amount of syntactic information that has to be processed in sentence construction. One group of patients tried to produce complete sentences using the entire amount of syntactic information, which distorted verb production. The other group attempted to make simple constructions. This made verbs easier to retrieve but led to sentences that were incomplete and objectless.

Acknowledgements

I thank the patients for their cooperation. Roelien Bastiaanse, Yosef Grodzinsky, Dirk-Bart den Ouden and Laura Sabourin are acknowledged for their helpful comments on an earlier draft of this article. This study was financially supported by the Foundation for Language, Speech and Logic, which is funded by the Netherlands Organization for Scientific Research (NWO).

Chapter 8
Effect of verb complexity on agrammatic aphasics' sentence production

KATALIN KISS

Introduction

The term 'agrammatism' covers different phenomena which are regarded as characteristic of Broca's aphasic language performance. The status of agrammatism as a 'natural category' or 'diagnostic class' has been heavily debated, nevertheless no researchers doubt the existence of agrammatic symptoms manifested in different language modalities (Badecker and Caramazza, 1985a, b; Caplan 1986, 1991; Miceli, Silveri, Romani and Caramazza, 1989). Agrammatism is a complex disorder encompassing several factors.

The most striking feature of agrammatism is the dysfunction of the ability to produce sentences or syntactic structures. Parallel to agrammatic sentence production many agrammatics show a syntactic deficit in language comprehension as well (Caramazza and Zurif, 1976; Schwartz, Saffran and Marin, 1980; Grodzinsky, 1984, 1986, 1990; Schwartz, Linebarger, Saffran and Pate, 1987; Linebarger, 1989,1990; Haarmann and Kolk, 1991, 1994; Mauner, Fromkin and Cornell, 1993; Hickok, Zurif and Canseco-Gonzalez, 1993; Zurif, Swinney, Prather, Solomon and Bushell, 1993; Frazier and McNamara, 1995; Swinney and Zurif, 1995; Kolk and Weijts, 1996). Using Thompson, Shapiro and Roberts' summary (1993) the deficit of sentence production can be characterized by the following main phenomena:

> reduction in the use of free and bound inflectional morphology; lack of grammatical agreement; 'telegraphic' style; reduction in the use of complex sentence structures (including passives, wh-questions, and relative clauses...; misordering of arguments (e.g. noun phrases) in sentence production...; a 'mapping' deficit...; and the deletion or mis-selection of terminal non-lexical elements (e.g. inflections, agreement, and complementizers in the phrasal geometry of a sentence...) (pp.111–12).

One part of the symptoms refers to the disorder of syntactic structure building processes. Construing simple active sentences agrammatic patients often produce fragments, incomplete DPs, prepositional phrases (PPs) and verb phrases (VPs) from which arguments and modifiers are lacking. Complex sentences or derived structures which are construed by movement (according to the Government and Binding (GB) Theory (Chomsky, 1981, 1986b)) are more vulnerable. The constituent movement factor contributes to the agrammatics' performance deficit (Kolk, 1995) because 'processing consequences of movement could constitute a computational load factor' (Kolk and Weijts, 1996: 112).

Assignment of superficial sentence features is also disturbed in agrammatic speech: case markers, verb inflectional endings, agreement morphemes, determiners and prefixes are often omitted or substituted. The omission of closed class elements can be interpreted in different ways. It can indicate that 'inflectional' and 'function word' components of morphological processing could form a functionally autonomous subcomponent of the lexicon. Selective damage of this subcomponent may be connected with disrupted information coming from the 'grammatical marker lexicon' or it could be related to the dysfunction of mechanisms responsible for assigning and interpreting syntactic features of sentences (Miceli, Silveri, Villa and Caramazza, 1984; Miceli and Caramazza, 1988).

In certain cases the 'form class component' of morphology seems to be disturbed separately. There are clinical data in the literature that describe a 'subtype' of agrammatic speech characterized by well-preserved use of word order and verb selection, and impaired use of inflections and function words (Tissot, Mounin, Lhermitte and Dordain, 1973). Miceli, Mazzuchi, Menn and Goodglass (1983) describe a patient who presented a severe deficit in grammatical marker production and retained his ability to select main verbs. Deep dyslexic patients (who often show agrammatic symptoms in their speech production) produce a high error rate reading isolated function words relative to content words (Coltheart, Patterson and Marshall, 1980). However, within the function word category much variance was found at deep dyslexic patients (De Bleser and Bayer, 1990).

The lexical deficit or morphological deficit account in itself does not seem to be sufficient to explain the impairment of grammatical marker production. It does not account for the diversity of agrammatics' formative production in different tasks: spontaneous speech samples are characterized by omission errors but in other elicitation tasks (picture description or connected speech) rather the substitution of grammatical morphemes was observed (Heeschen,1985; Kolk and Heeschen, 1992). Omission rate or the proportion of function words can vary, even in the same patient's speech (Bastiaanse, 1995). In richly inflected languages, like Italian, substitution of closed class elements is more common than omission errors (Bates, Friederici and Wulfeck, 1987).

The problem of formatives can be explained from a syntactic aspect supposing that a syntactic deficit has consequences for the production of grammatical morphology (Kolk, 1995). If the syntactic component does not produce a full phrase structure representation (syntactic frame with categorized slots) during the initial structure building the sentence structure could not be interpreted coherently on a later processing stage. Functional categories cannot create a functional relation with the relevant units if the sentence production system does not deliver these nodes or slots at a given point in time. For example, case is assigned under Government according to the GB Theory. Government is a constraint in the model of grammar that identifies the structural relation between the governor and governed constituents. This configurational condition can not be fulfilled if the slot of the governing head and the slot of the XP to which the case is assigned are not presented simultaneously in the syntactic frame. Production of a closed class morpheme or the assignment of thematic roles is possible, as soon as the minimally required structural representation is available (Kolk, 1995; Kolk and Weijts, 1996). Thematic relations cannot take place, the Theta Criterion could not be fulfilled if the initial syntactic frame is incomplete or incompatible with the subcategorization requirement of the given verb.

Sentence formation and parsing of sentences presuppose the interaction of subsystems of the lexicon with modules of grammar.

Construction of a simple sentence presumes different cognitive mechanisms operating simultaneously or successively: verb processing, activation of verb information e.g. access to the subcategorization list and predicate–argument structure, thematic role assignment to argument noun phrases (NPs); construction of the base sentence structure according to the phrase structure rules of the given language; semantic selection/lexical access of elements belonging to different syntactic categories and assigning syntactic features e.g. overt case, verb tense, agreement.

Agrammatic aphasics who are native speakers of typologically different languages produce various kinds of symptoms in sentence production which can be explained by the parametric differences of their languages. Deficiency of syntactic operation of thematic role assignment, for example, can manifest itself in a word order disorder or misordering of arguments in English, but in Hungarian misordering of arguments is not relevant as different permutations of the major constituents of the sentence can be equally grammatical. It is rather the deletion/substitution or misinterpretation of case markers that signs the 'mapping deficit' in Hungarian agrammatics' verbal output and sentence comprehension as the syntactic function of constituents is marked non-configurationally, by overt case markers. The case suffix marks that an NP behaves as a thematic role bearing argument in the phrase structure.

Assuming that the sentence processing system is composed of two basic subsystems, a syntactic and a thematic processor (Rayner, Carlson and Frazier, 1983; Tanenhaus, Carlson and Trueswell, 1989), agrammatics can fail to produce simple sentences if they activate only partial information from the lexical entry of the verb (e.g. verb-based thematic information and argument structure) or if they are not able to construct full structural representations.

In this study we investigate how Hungarian Broca's aphasic patients can lexically select and retrieve verbs which differ in their representational complexities and how are they able to construe VPs and simple sentences using the target predicate. The aim of the examination was to investigate verb production but it is evident that we can not speak about verb processing as a separate function from simple sentence structure formation.

As the elicitation task an off-line method, a 'picture description/action naming' test was used; the data were interpreted in the theoretical framework of GB Theory.

Hungarian sentence structure

Hungarian is an agglutinating Finno-Ugric language (like Finnish, Estonian, Samoyed and Vogul).

Inflectional suffixes of the finite verb indicate tense or mood, they express number and person of the subject and (in)definiteness of the object NP. The finite verb's suffix is in agreement with the suffix of subject NP in person and number.

The syntactic functions of sentence constituents are expressed by case markers (suffixes) on the argument nouns. There are at least 17 cases and 38 morpho-phonological variants of surface case-ending forms in Hungarian (Antal, 1977).

Among the proposed sentence structure models of Hungarian (Horvath, 1986; Brody, 1990; Marácz, 1990) we introduce the analysis of É. Kiss (1987, 1990, 1994a).

Hungarian sentence structure divides into a topic and a VP. The topic serves as a logical or notional subject, the VP serves as the logical predicate of the sentence.

According to É. Kiss the sentence is not the projection of a functional category but is the instantiation of a predication relation. In her later work É. Kiss assumes that the sentence is projected from the functional category of tense or mood (see É. Kiss, 1995).

In É. Kiss's model all the arguments of the verb are generated VP-internally in an arbitrary order. All arguments are sisters, the subject and the object are structurally parallel.

In Hungarian the syntactic function of constituents does not play a role in the sentence structure hierarchy, the subject does not have a prominent

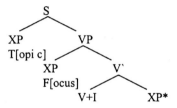

Figure 8.1. Phrase structure of Hungarian. XP* = the verb's obligatory and facultative arguments: NP/DP, PP (post-position phrase).

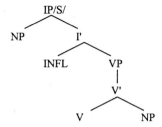

Figure 8.2. Phrase structure of English.

position. The hierarchy of predicate–argument relations cannot be identified through relations in the phrase structure (in English the relationship between phrase structure and lexical structure can be described by identity).

In configurational languages like English the subject and object behave differently because of their positional asymmetry in the sentence structure hierarchy. The subject is in a higher position – dominated by the S-node – than the object which is dominated by the VP node. The object receives its Theta-role from the V whereas the subject is Theta marked by the VP (Chomsky, 1981, 1986b). Others hypothesized that the subject is also Theta assigned locally in the VP then moves up to [Spec, IP] position binding a trace in [Spec, VP] [VP-Internal Subject Hypothesis (Woolford, 1991)].

The primary function of the English phrase structure is to encode the syntactic function of the constituent NPs. In Hungarian case markers provide this function. Case assignment, including nominative assignment, takes place in the VP, because the tense and agreement morphemes, which are dominated by the I(nflection), are lowered on to the V (É. Kiss, 1994b).

The different constituent orders of the Hungarian sentence can be produced by two transformation rules: topicalization and focusing, and by parallely used stress rules. (It is not obligatory to fill in the topic and focus position.)

Topicalization is a movement rule which preposes an XP from the [XP, V'] position to the [XP, S] position. The topic position can be filled with an unstressed maximal category (including null), multiple topics are created by adjunction to S. The topic functions semantically as a notional subject about which the VP predicates something. The VP bears a primary predication relation to the topicalized XP: they mutually m-command each other and the topicalized XP binds an empty argument position in the VP. In neutral sentences each major constituent bears identical stress.

In 'non-neutral' sentences that contain focused category the immediately preverbal position [Spec, VP] is filled in with a primary (heavy) stressed maximal category extracted from the [XP, V'] position. The verb itself also can be focused. Focusing is a *Wh* movement type of transformation: it moves a constituent from argument position into an operator position from which the moved constituent c-commands its scope. Focus operator serves to express identification which goes together with exclusion (contrast) when the focus operates on a closed set of individuals.

An SVO string in Hungarian can be differently interpreted according to the intonational pattern of the SVO sentence:

1. (TopicVO) neutral sentence: *János kergette a macskát. – John chased the cat* or
2. (FocusVO) contrastive sentence: *"János kergette a macskát – It is John who chased the cat* (" : marks focus stress)
3. non-neutral sentence with heavy stress on the verb: *János "kergette a macskát. – John DID chase the cat* (emphatic sentence) or *What John actually did to the cat was chasing it* – rather than feeding, for example [(SFocusO) contrastive sentence]

A sentence of SOV order can be interpreted as

1. (SFocusV) contrastive sentence: *János a "macskát kergette – Actually, it is the cat that John chased.*
2. (TTV) neutral sentence with multiple topic: *János a macskát kergette – /John-nom. the cat-acc. chased/ John chased the cat.*
3. *SOV sentence with unquantified common noun in the preverbal modifier position János levelet írt. – /* John-*nom. letter-acc. wrote/ – John was letter-writing.*

The order of words in phrases, e.g. in possessive DP, in postpositional and adjective phrases are fixed in Hungarian. The order of verb and argument NPs are free but operators like focus, WH operator and negated constituent have to land in VP-peripheral positions, quantifiers are left-adjoined to VP. Predicate adverbials are dominated by the VP, sentential adverbials are dominated by the S-node (they can take place before or after the topic, or between topics).

Verb processing in agrammatism

Since the 1980s several studies have examined agrammatic aphasics' ability to produce verb phrases and process verb information. Results from different types of elicitation tasks demonstrate that verb retrieval is significantly more impaired than noun retrieval in agrammatic aphasics. Agrammatics show a marked deficit in naming actions, verbs are underrepresented in their spontaneous speech, verb inflection and auxiliaries are also affected (Saffran, Schwartz and Marin, 1980; Miceli, Silveri, Villa and Caramazza, 1984; McCarthy and Warrington, 1985; Zingeser and Berndt, 1990; Marshall, Pring and Chiat, 1993). The reduced proportion of verbs in agrammatic output raises the question whether the difficulty of producing main verbs and grammatical markers is closely or accidentally related. Does the tendency to omit verbs imply a lexical or a syntactic processing deficit in agrammatism (Miceli, Silveri, Villa and Caramazza, 1984)? Several other studies focused on the role of verbs in sentence comprehension. Schwartz, Saffran and Marin (1980) examined word-order impairment in English Broca's aphasics using simple active declarative sentences involving two-place predicates (like The horse kicks the cow). Recognition of the syntactic functions of the argument NPs in these sentences was based on the interpretation of information manifest in the surface word order. Agrammatic aphasics failed to analyse the basic relational structure of the sentences or to decode the syntactic relations because of a dysfunction of those processes which map/assign the thematic roles on to the grammatical categories, e.g. to subject, direct-object argument NPs. Other results also confirmed that agrammatics' inability to interpret certain structures could be explained by the deficit of a 'mapping' procedure (Linebarger, Schwartz and Saffran, 1983; Schwartz, Linebarger, Saffran and Pate,1987; Caramazza and Miceli, 1991).

When normal syntactic parsing operations are disturbed, agrammatic patients use alternative ways in the semantic interpretation of the sentence. Broca's aphasics show 'at chance or below chance' performance in the comprehension of passive sentences, they misinterpret the thematic role of the subject NP. A passive verb has one internal argument to which it assigns the Theme thematic role directly. Because the passive verb cannot assign accusative to the Theme, the latter argument moves to the subject position to get nominative case from the finite I, leaving a trace in its original (complement) position. The thematic role of the subject NP can be identified only across the trace that is co-indexed with the NP. Agrammatics show difficulty in semantic interpretation if the thematic role assignment is mediated by a trace. If the mechanism of co-indexation fails, the NP cannot bind the trace therefore their referencial-dependency can not be established (Mauner, 1993). Grodzinsky (1984, 1986) in his Trace

Deletion Hypothesis assumes that S-structure representation lacks traces therefore the thematic role information of the subject NP is disrupted. The patients use 'heuristics' in the semantic interpretation of the sentence, like 'the sentence initial NP is usually the subject of the sentence' or 'the subject NP is usually Agent'. Using this alternative strategy agrammatics associate the Agent role to the moved NP. Because the preposition 'by' in the adjunct PP most frequently assigns the role of Agent to its sister NP, Broca's aphasics choose the Agent randomly.

In Hungarian, morphological case marking was found to play the leading role in the interpretation of syntactic relations in a comprehension test. Hungarian aphasics decoded the unmarked (nominative) NP as Agent/subject in simple sentences which involved transitive verbs, but in those cases when the case markers were removed, tendency was found to interpret the NVN strings as SVO and the NNV string as SOV structures (MacWhinney and Osman-Sági, 1991). This means that the case marker is a strong cue in the sentence interpretation.

The syntactic complexity of verbs seems to be another decisive factor in decoding or generating sentences both in normal and agrammatic persons.

Saffran, Schwartz and Marin (1980) observed that agrammatic aphasics have more problems in understanding verbs with two or three arguments than in decoding those verbs which assign only one Agent/subject participant (e.g. follow, push away vs. smile, cry).

Shapiro, Zurif and Grimshaw (1987) investigated the effect of the 'representational' complexity of verbs in normal speakers' sentence comprehension and found that the amount of representation information affects the sentence processing. They examined verbs that differed from each other in their 'subcategorization complexities' and 'argument structure complexities' (verbs that allow one or more subcategorization and argument structure possibilities).[1]

The following order of verb difficulty was determined on the basis of reaction times (RT) in a Cross-Modal Lexical Decision Task (CMLD):

transitive < non-alternating dative = alternating dative = two complement < four complement.

The authors concluded that a verb's potential for different thematic structures seemed to be a relevant factor for the sentence processing complexity. The non-alternating and alternating dative verbs did not yield significant differences in RT because their argument structures were the same even though they allowed different syntactic subcategorization possibilities. In the group of 'four complement' verbs longer RT were observed compared to the 'two complement' group. Even though both verb types select the same subcategorization frame the 'four complement' verbs allow more 'semantic types' (P, Q, I); that is 'the relevant verb complexity metric for sentence processing involves the argument structure of verbs and not the syntactic subcategorization' (Shapiro, Zurif and Grimshaw, 1987: 241).

In the second part of their experiment Shapiro et al. investigated the 'argument structure complexity' effect with respect to the role of optional (implicit) vs. obligatory arguments. The data showed that verbs allowing only one argument structure arrangement (transitive and obligatory three-place predicates, like *to hand*) did not differ significantly in contrast to those types of verbs that allowed both a two-place and an optional three-place argument structure (alternating and non-alternating dative verbs). This suggested that 'the crucial metric for sentence processing complexity is the number of possible argument structure arrangements not the number of arguments within a given arrangement' (Shapiro, Zurif and Grimshaw, 1987: 241). Investigating agrammatic Broca's aphasics with the above-mentioned test materials and method, Shapiro and Levin (1990) found that agrammatic aphasics showed the same RT pattern as the normal subjects in both CMLD probes. The authors concluded that the device that activates the verb and its structural properties operates normally during sentence comprehension in Broca's aphasics. The difficulties observed in the understanding of complex structures (passives, relative clauses) thus arise from the dysfunction of the post-activation processing which is responsible for the assignment of thematic roles to argument NPs.

Other experimental results showed that mis-selection of a special semantic feature assigned in the semantic representation of the verb could also result in a thematic role assignment deficit which could be manifested in argument reversing.

Jones (1984) found that understanding sentences containing 'directional motion verbs' (e.g. *follow, push, pull*) was significantly more difficult for agrammatic aphasics than processing sentences containing 'non-motion verbs'. The directional motion verb has a special semantic property which alone determines the relationship of the arguments. These verbs involve 'inherent embedded prepositions' that specify a directional/spatial relation between their (Agent-Theme/Patient) arguments. Misinterpretation of the perceptual feature of the verb (direction expressed by the inner preposition: e.g. follow ((NP1 NP2) [MOTION, NP1 **before** NP2]) causes a 'mental reversing' which presents itself in an argument misordering (e.g. instead of *The man follows the girl* > *The girl follows the man*).

In our unpublished material (Kiss, Mészáros and Kiefer, 1992) we observed the same phenomena in aphasics' verbal output (using an action description test where the actions were presented on video). The 'place-coordinates' of the directional motion verbs were often inverted, the directional features ('moving away' or 'approaching') were switched which resulted in verb substitutions (e.g. *The girl is pushing the car into the garage* > *She is pulling it*). In the case of three-place predicates which take 'dative' complements, the 'converse approach' was also observed. The verb substitution was caused by replacing the Agent (Giver) and Benefactive (Receiver) roles (e.g. *The girl gives the plate to the boy* > *The boy takes the plate from the girl*). A similar 'converse approach' was found in the case of two-place causative verbs when the aphasic patients often approached the event not from the viewpoint of the Agent but from that of the Patient. This resulted in the deletion of the obligatory accusative argument and as a result of 'decausativation' an active intransitive verb was used (e.g. *he makes the horse jump* > *it is jumping*). The converse approach seems to be a compensation strategy in the case of causatives because the 'change of perspective' gives the possibility of selecting a less complex verb which could be more easily retrieved.

The above data show that some typical Broca's aphasic phenomena are closely related to the dysfunction of verb processing.

Representation of verbs

Because verbs have a critical role in sentence planning processes, we can assume a causal connection between disorder of sentence production and dysfunction of verb retrieval in agrammatics. The lexical-semantic information specified in the lexical entry of the verb determines the relations of the minimal constituents in a sentence. According to GB Theory (Chomsky, 1981, 1986a, b), each verb has selection properties which are represented in the mental lexicon via the 'subcategorization frame' and the 'argument structure'. Subcategorization (category selection property) is a restriction between the verb and the syntactic category of its complements, the semantic selection entails a restriction between the predicate and the semantic types of its complements. Every complement of the verb must be semantically selected.

The subcategorization frame of the verb involves the list of complements which are obligatory constituents of the verb phrase. A verb subcategorizes for a complement if it is lexically governed by the verb. The form of the complements can be different: NP, PP, S' (sentential clause) or combinations of these phrases. Some verbs allow more subcategorization alternations, e.g. the verb *carry* or *believe*. Other verbs, like *meet*, have only one subcategorization possibility.

The predicate–argument structure and thematic information are also part of the lexical entry of the verb. The arguments are those NPs to which thematic roles are assigned by the verb. The thematic roles like Agent, Theme, Goal are certain types of semantic/conceptual information which define specific semantic relationships between the verb and its arguments (Jackendoff, 1972). The thematic roles must be assigned to the arguments which have to be realized structurally in an appropriate syntactic position. Each verb selects its arguments and assigns them thematic roles idiosyncratically. Some verbs like *send* or *buy* allow two types of realization of their arguments: a two-place (x, y) and a three-place (x, y, z) structure.

3.   *send*   a-structure: (x, y)
                                        (x, y, z)
              thematic grid   (Agent, Theme)
                                     (Agent, Theme, Goal)

The Goal argument can be regarded as an 'implicit' argument because its structural realization is optional. Other verbs like *to hand* are obligatory three-place verbs, their third Goal arguments must always be realized syntactically.

Because strict subcategorization is relevant to syntax (it imposes well-formedness conditions on a syntactic level) and semantic selection is relevant both to semantics and syntax, the representational complexity of a predicate has an effect on the generation of simple sentences in agrammatic aphasics.

In this study we investigated the role of verb complexity in the semantic selection and syntactic processes using verbs of different argument structure complexities with different morphological complexities. We concentrated on the question of what kind of information is attainable from the lexical representation of a verb and what kind of operations and mechanisms are used in the syntactic structure building processes if the lexical accessibility of the verb is disturbed.

The structure of the verbs used in the present study

Based on their argument structure complexities, the tested verbs of the present study formed three main groups. **Group I** involves one-place intransitive predicates which take only one Agent or Experient argument. **Group II** involves two-place verbs, **Group III** involves three-place predicates.

Each main verb group is represented by several subgroups.

Group I/A contains morphologically and semantically simple one-place verbs (S), e.g. *alszik* (sleep), *ásít* (yawn).

Group I/B contains one-place reflexive verbs (R) e.g. *borotválkozik* (shave oneself), *zuhanyozik* (take a shower), *vakarózik* (scratch oneself), *nyújtózkodik* (stretch oneself). These types of reflexives assign an 'inner' Patient (Theme) argument. Because it is only an 'inner' argument, syntactic function does not belong to it, it cannot be mapped into an overt object NP. The inner Patient argument is identified by the semantic representation of the predicate, the Patient is identical with the Agent (Komlósy, 1994), e.g.

4.   *fésülködik*   semantic representation: 'x   *fésüli*   y-t   x = y'
     (comb oneself)   ('x-nom combs y-acc.')

Reflexives are morphologically complex because they are derived from a verb stem by reflexive suffix.

Group I/C contains one-place verbs which are derived from a noun by a denominal derivational suffix (N>V) e.g. *teniszezik* (play tennis), *síel* (ski), *csónakázik* (boat).

The derived predicates in Group C contain an 'atomic predicate' in their semantic representation, like 'MOVE/GO', 'PLAY', 'USE', which assign the original noun stems as argument. Because of word formation/derivation these complements become 'inner' semantic arguments, they are not expressed syntactically but are identified by the semantic representation of the derived predicate (Jackendoff, 1987; Komlósy, 1994). The derived verb *'gitározik'* for example, has the following semantic representation:

5. *gitározik*
    'plays the guitar': *Morphological form:*
                         gitár   - ozik
                         stem   suffix

                         Semantic representation:
                         JÁTSZIK   *a*   *gitáron*
                         PLAY-3sg   the   guitar-on
                         [atomic predicate]   [inner argument]
                         '(he) plays the guitar'

Table 8.1. Main features of the verbs in Group I

	I/A simple		I/B reflexive		I/C N>V	
Syntactic complexity	*sír* 'cry'	(x) (Agent)	*fésülködik* 'comb oneself'	(x) (Agent)	*gitározik* 'play the guitar'	(x) (Agent)
Morphological complexity	—		stem + **-kozik/közik/kôzik -kodik/ködik -ózik,-ódzik** reflexive suffix		noun stem + **-z(ik)** **-l/al/el** derivational suffix	
Semantic complexity	—		'inner' Patient arg.		'inner' argument	

Group II contains three subgroups:

Group II/A contains *reversible transitive predicates*: the Theme argument is mapped to an object NP in which the noun is specified as [+animate].

6. *megvigasztal* ('comfort')   [NPnom., NPacc.]
    A   *férfi*   *megvigasztalja*   *a*   *lányt.*
    the   man-nom.   prefix-comfort-3sg.def. the   girl-acc.
    'The man comforts the girl.'

Group II/B contains irreversible transitive verbs: there is animacy contrast between the Agent and Patient/Theme arguments, the Theme/Patient-object argument has [–animate] semantic features.

7. *hámoz*　　　('peel')　　　　[NPnom, NPacc]
　 A　　　　*fiú*　　　　　*meghámozza*　　　　　　　*a*　　*banánt.*
　 the　　　　boy-nom.　　prefix-peel-3sg.indef.　　the　banana-acc
　 'The boy peels the banana.'

Group II/C contains predicates that assign an Agent thematic role to the subject and Goal/Source/Location thematic role to their locative arguments.

8. *átmegy*　　　('cross')　　　[NPnom, NPsuperess.]
　 A　　　　*férfi*　　　*átmegy*　　　　　　*az*　　*úttesten*
　 the　　　　man　　　across-go-3sg.　　the　　road-on
　 'The man is crossing the road.'

Group III contains two subgroups:
　　Group III/A contains verbs that assign Agent-Theme-Goal/Source/ Location thematic roles which have to be mapped into the subject, object and locative NPs.

9. *beletesz*　　　　('put into')　　　[NPnom, NPacc, NP illative]
　 A　*férfi*　　*beteszi*　　　*a*　　*böröndöt*　*az*　*autóba.*
　 the　man-nom.　into-put-3sg.def.　the　suitcase-acc.　the　car-into
　 'The man puts the suitcase into the car.'

Group III/B contains verbs that assign Agent-Theme-Benefactive/Goal thematic roles, requiring subject, object and dative complements.

10. *bemutat*　　　('introduce')　　　　[NPnom., NPacc., NP dat.]
　 A　*fiú*　　*bemutatja*　　　*a*　*lányt*　*a*　*barátjának.*
　 the　boy-nom.　prefix-introduce-3sg-def.　the　girl-acc　the　friend-
　　　　　　　　　　　　　　　　　　　　　　　　　　　　gen-3sg-dat.
　 'The boy introduces the girl to his friend.'

Method

Subjects

The verbal performance of two agrammatic Broca's aphasic patients was analysed. Both patients are native speakers of Hungarian.

　　A.N. A 55-year-old, female, right-handed nurse (education: secondary school) was rehospitalized 20 month post-onset when deterioration was observed in her condition, as a result of a second cerebrovascular insult.

L.I. A 37-year-old, female, right-handed radiological assistant (education: specialized matriculation examination) was investigated 36 months post-onset.

Both patients suffered a left lateral cerebro-vascular accident and had right hemiparesis. CT scans for A.N. showed previous parieto-occipital involvement and frontal hypodensity which was the sign of a second, acute vascular lesion. L.I.'s CT scan showed large temporo-parieto-occipital hypodensity which signalled a middle cerebral artery and posterior artery infarct. Classification of aphasia type was made by the Hungarian Variant of the Western Aphasia Battery (Osman-Sági, 1991). (A.N.'s WAB AQ:49; L.I.'s WAB AQ: 65.4.)

A.N.'s spontaneous speech showed reduced fluency, telegraphic style and severe speech initiation difficulty, it hardly contained intact propositions or sentences. Her speech consisted of automatic, stereotyped phrases, isolated words and paraphasias.

Spontaneous speech sample of A.N.:

> 'Istenem! ... Beteg voltam ... Marika ... Nem tudom ... kórház ... professzor ... Szent János Kórház ... Jó napot, óó, nem nem! ... Ó Istenem! ... Nem tudok ... Beszéd ... Nem ...'
>
> ('Oh, my God! ... I was ill ... Mary ... I do not know ... hospital ... professor ... St John Hospital ... Good morning, oh no, no! ... Oh God! ... I cannot ... Speech ... No ...')

After a 3-month therapy period she showed some improvement according to the Western test (WAB AQ: 54.6), but the character of her spontaneous speech did not really change. She was tested with the 'action description test' at the beginning of therapy and 3 months later. In the present study we analysed her answers given in both of the 'action naming tests'.

L.I.'s spontaneous speech was also non-fluent, characterized by marked anomia and agrammatic symptoms. She often used more automatic speech 'panels' or expressions, e.g. 'I knew that something is wrong', 'I am fed up', 'It was evening when it happened', 'I could not do anything'. She filled in the hesitation gaps caused by word-finding difficulties with these grammatically well-formed phrases and with some adverbs. She was able to use active non-stereotype simple clauses but she had difficulty producing complex sentences. She produced many incomplete phrases (VPs and DPs as well) or sentences (with often incomplete subordinate clauses). Semantic selection and access problem of the 'lexical verbs' was an outstanding symptom in her speech; the type/token ratio of verbs was relatively low in her spontaneous speech, she retrieved mostly modal verbs (e.g. must, can, ought, might) and she often used the verb 'know'. Omission and morphological errors of verb inflection and case marking of nouns were also observed.

Speech sample of L.I.:

'L.I.: Lehet, hogyha valami vé végett kellene úszni, aa..akkor lehet, hogy jó lenne, de ... most most nem. És és nem nem tudok. Olyan olyan nem félsz ... Csak csak olyan ... olyan elegem van és és nem tudok. Mindegy, hát ez ... Therapist: És mit sportolt még?

L.I.: Énnekem? Ajaj! ... Egy vi vitorlázó ... gépet ... Hát a zzzzzz ...

T: Repülô? Vitorlázó repülô?

L.I.: Igen! Dehát a anyám a azt mondta, hogy...hogy nem. Nem lehet, mert ...

T: Mert?

L.I.: Hát hát a szülôk ... nem ... nem ... Tudják, hogy hogy lehet, hogy valami baj van, vagy ... dehát az ... De de az az az jó volt.'

(L.I.: Maybe if it should ... sw ... swimm ... because because of something, then ... then ... maybe it would be OK but ... now ... now not. And and I cannot cannot. Like like you do not fear /not fear/... It is it is like ... like I am fed up and and I cannot. It does not matter, well this ...

T: And what kind of other sport did you do?

L.I.: For me? Huu! ... A gli ... a glider ... Well a zzzzzz ...

T: A plane? A glider?

L.I.: Yes! But my mother told me, that ... that no. It is impossible because ...

T: Because?

L.I.: Because the parents ... no, no ... They know that that it can happen that something is wrong or ... but that ... But but that that that was good.)

Material

The test material contained 124 target verbs which belonged to eight verb types (Group I/A–C, II/A–C, III/A, B, as described above). Our elicitation method was an 'action naming' /'picture description' test. The pictures that represented the target verbs/actions were assembled from Jacqueline Stark: 'Everyday Life Activities (photo series)' collection (Stark, 1992). Each coloured photocard of the series represents one particular action.

Procedure

The subjects were tested individually, the photocards were randomly presented one after another. The aphasics were instructed to describe or tell us 'what happened in the picture', who the actors were, what they were doing. (The patients were asked to imagine describing the picture to someone who is also in the room who does not see the picture, therefore they should try to give as precise a description as possible or as they can.) Responses were tape-recorded and transcribed. General help like 'Could you tell me anything more?', phonemic cues (whispering of first syllable), questions referring to an argument noun or supplying of an argument noun were used only when the patients asked for help. In the statistical analysis we used only the independent, spontaneous answers.

Results

Table 8.2 shows the proportions of the verbs produced by the aphasics according to different types of predicates and the distribution of the complete, grammatically well-formed sentences involving the target verbs. We regarded an answer to be 'complete' if the patients were able to build the whole VP or sentence. It means that the verb and its complements were lexically accessible, the argument NPs were supplied with the appropriate overt case marker, noun–verb agreement was intact and non-terminal node deletion did not occur. If an inflectional or a derivational ending or a determiner was omitted or any argument was missing we did not accept the incomplete clause as a 'correct' response even if the verb retrieval itself was successful e.g.

* *Nem kártya. Fiúnak odaadta.* (Not card-nom. Boy-dat. prefix-give-3sg.def.past)
* *Önteni önteni a limonádét.*(To pour to pour the lemonade-acc).
* *Doktornô, doktor megvizsgálja.*(Doctoress-nom, doctor-nom examine-3sg.def.)
* *Nézeget az óra.* (Look-frequent.suff-3sg.indef the clock-nom.)

Because Hungarian is a pro-drop language, the subject pronoun may be left unexpressed. If there is no overt subject NP in the sentence the Agent role is assigned to a phonetically empty pronoun (*pro*). The verb inflection refers to the number and person of the subject (in the case of the target verbs it was the third-person singular form). We accepted those answers as 'complete clauses' in which the aphasics did not assign an overt subject NP but used the right inflected verb form e.g. *'Felébreszti a fiút'* ((pro) wake-3sg.def. up the boy-acc.).

Predicates 'precisely' described the action represented in the given picture constitute the **target** verbs. Verb **substitutions** contain irrelevant responses or verbs which do not 'exactly' express the given action although they are adequate to the situational context e.g.

target verb: *The man* goes upstairs. > substituted verb: *'he is* sitting'
target verb: *The boy* wipes the milk. > substituted verb: *'he* spills'
target verb: *The girl* wakes up the boy. > substituted verb: *'he is* sleeping'
target verb: *The man* kisses the women. > substituted verb: *'he* loves her '
target verb: *The man* puts the suitcase into the car. > substituted verb: *'mum* packs up'

The analysis of the data shows that the mean scores of the complete clauses were much higher in the 'one-place' verb group (39.6) than with the 'two-place' (3.8) or 'three-place' (6.3) predicates. In the latter two groups the ratios of complete clauses were very low.

Table 8.2. Disribution of complete clauses and verbs (percentage values are in parentheses)

	One-place			Two-place			Tree-place	
	I/A simple	I/B reflex.	I/C N/V	II/A [+anim]	II/B [–anim]	II/C locative	III/A locative	III/B dative
Number of target verbs	12	9	21	15	35	11	13	8
Total no. of responses	36	27	63	45	105	33	39	24
Complete clauses	26 (72.2)	8 (29.6)	16 (25.3)	2 (4.4)	5 (4.7)	0 (0)	1 (2.5)	3 (12.5)
Mean score of complete clauses	(39.6)			(3.8)			(6.3)	
Target verb	26 (72.2)	8 (29.6)	16 (25.3)	11 (24.4)	24 (22.8)	0 (0)	4 (10.2)	4 (16.6)
Verb substitut.	5	7	6	29	41	25	20	15
Total verb responses	31 (86.1)	15 (55.5)	22 (31.7)	40 (88.8)	65 (61.9)	25 (75.9)	24 (61.5)	19 (79.1)
Mean of total verb responses	(54.8)			(71.0)			(66.6)	

Not surprisingly, constructing a surface sentence which involved a one-place predicate was easier for the agrammatic aphasics than constructing a syntactic structure which contained a two- or three-place verb. If the patient was able to access the one-place predicate, she could also construct the whole VP. In the case of the two- and three-place predicates, however, retrieval of the verb's phonetic form did not mean a simultaneously successful syntactic structure building. The construction of the surface sentence was perfect for roughly one-quarter of those answers which contained the target verb. This phenomenon shows a mapping disorder, the patients are limited in the 'monitoring' of the assignment of multiple arguments into the appropriate slots of the syntactic frame.

Comparing the distribution of the retrievable target verbs within each verb group we found the following 'verb difficulty order':

simple one-place > morphologically complex one-place (R and N>V) = transitive (two-place) > three-place (with locative and dative complement) > two-place with locative complement

Access to the 'simple one-place' verbs was outstandingly successful (72.2).

The lexical selection of the 'two-place verbs with locative complement' proved to be the most difficult for the patients (they could not retrieve any verb in this group). These predicates were directional motion verbs. The lexical representations of these verbs integrate mental knowledge related to the cognitive representation of space or spatial relations. These verbs include such contents as direction of the motion, place-coordinates, starting point and end point. This information is encoded in the semantic representation and thematic roles of the predicate. Processing of this information seemed to be more difficult for our patients, they produced marked selection disorder when attempting to produce these verbs.

We did not find large differences in the proportion of activated verbs among the 'one-place reflexive' (29.6), 'one-place derived from noun' (25.3) and 'two-place transitive' (24.4; 22.8) verb groups. Proportions of these verbs were lower in contrast to the 'simple one-place verb' group.

The ratios of the three-place verbs (10.2;16.6) were lower than the proportions of the one-place and two-place verbs (except the 'two-place locative' group).

The results show that the 'representational complexity' of the predicate has a direct effect on the lexical accessibility of the verb for agrammatic aphasics. The argument-structure complexity of the verb (number of obligatory arguments) plays an important role in verb retrieval but it is not the only factor. The morphological and semantic representational complexity of the 'one-place derived verbs' (I/B, I/C) and the semantic representational complexity of the 'two-place locative' verbs also had an effect on the lexical-semantic selection of the predicates.

In the next part of the study we would like to present some further data which refer to particular 'tendencies' or 'strategies' observed in the aphasic patients' performance. These tendencies were outlined during 'error analysis'. (We need further investigation and more data to interpret these results more precisely.)

Effects of morphological complexity

In the Group I/C two types of answers were found which were related to the morphological structure of the verb:

a. **noun stem (only)**
b. verbs: **– noun stem > target verb derivation**
                                 – target verb
                                 – verb substitution

The noun stem appeared in more than half of the answers, which means that the noun stem was activated first in many cases and it was used as 'access code' or 'mediator' in the retrieval process of the derived verb form, if the direct semantic access to the verb was not possible. The patients used an indirect retrieval method for the predicate by activating morphological processes/word formation rules. The noun stem was assigned first both in cases where the stem and derived form were regular and in those where they were not, e.g. *ló* > *lovagol* ('horse > ride the horse'). This strategy was found both in independent answers and in answers given by phonemic cue.

The data show that morphological complexity of the verb is a decisive representational factor that has an effect on the accessibility of the verb.

Table 8.3. Proportion of answers belonging to the different types

N stem	22.22
N stem > target V	30.15
Target V*	44.44
Substituted V	3,17

* The number of the target verb answers is higher here than in Table 8.2 because those answers which were not accepted as 'correct' were also considered during 'error analysis' that is, answers given by phonemic cue, infinitives, morphologically ill-formed forms.

Types of answers

In this part we analyse the different types of answers given by the subjects in the two- and three-place verb groups. In the analysis of the data three kinds of answer types were distinguished (see Appendix 8.1 for examples).

Type A. **Isolated argument/s** – activation of one argument or list of arguments (N or DP, case marked or caseless forms)

Type B. **Argument/s assignment** > followed by **Verb selection / Clausal answer** (involving the target or substituted/paraphasia verbs which were one-place or two-place predicates)

Type C. **Clausal answers** (no previous argument N or DP assignment)

Type D. **Other**: e.g. *'I don't know'* answer, noun associations. (In the further analysis these answers were not included.) These answers were rare 12/372 total answers.

The data show that our subjects had a lexical selection problem in accessing target predicates; they selected a high number of paraphasia verbs. Proportions of target verbs were lower than substituted verbs in every verb group.

This does not mean that the aphasic patients cannot obtain any information from the feature structure of the verbs. The unsuccessful retrieval of the phonological form of the target verb does not explain agrammatic verbal performance in itself. The argument 'enumerations' indicate that certain information concerning the argument-structure, thematic grid and subcategorization list is available.

Table 8.4. Distribution of answers in the 'A–C' types and distribution of target and substituted verbs in clauses

	II/A Two-place [+animate]	II/B Two-place [−animate]	II/C Two-place (locative)	III/A Three-place (locative)	III/B Three-place (dative)
Total no. of answers	45	96	30	38	23
Total no. of clausal answers	40	65	25	24	19
Type A	11.1	32.2	16.6	36.8	17.3
Type B	28.8	39.5	43.3	52.6	43.4
Type C	60.0	28.1	40.0	10.5	39.1
Target verb	27.5	36.9	0	16.7	21.1
Substitut. for one-place V	40.0	24.6	76.0	29.1	42.1
Substitut. for two-place V	32.5	38.5	24.0	54.1	36.8

In **Type A** answers only nouns or noun phrases were produced, the verb was deleted. In **Type B** answers the activation of nominal elements of the subcategorization list preceded lexical access of the verb. (During the selection of argument nouns hesitation, pauses, semantic paraphasias, word initiation difficulties, self-corrections occurred.) The subjects usually attempted to build the previously activated argument Ns or DPs into a syntactic scheme. When the phonetic form of the target verb was inaccessible, another predicate was selected (both one- or two-place verbs which were always adequate in the situational context).

Type C (and clausal part of **Type B**) answers were either fragments/agrammatic or well-formed sentences.

The 'listed' Ns or DPs (in 'isolated argument' answer types) were always complements, never randomly named nouns. (Instrument and locative adjunct NPs sometimes occurred.) The patients never assigned 'extra' arguments, only those which were required by the verb.

The data show that the subjects were able to get some specific information represented in the lexical entry of the predicate: argument-structure and thematic information were accessible; argument assignment was not accidental, the ratio of activated arguments with different thematic roles was related to the thematic hierarchy.

Argument assignment and thematic hierarchy

According to the Projection Principle of GB Theory, lexical information is syntactically represented. Argument structure is projected from the lexical semantic structure of the verb and the base structure of the sentence is projected from the argument structure according to the parametric characteristics of phrase structure of a given language (Grimshaw, 1990).

According to the 'thematic hierarchy' hypothesis, the argument structure of the verb is not only a set of arguments. It has its own internal structure which represents prominent relations that are determined by the thematic information of the predicate (Grimshaw, 1990). Grimshaw suggested a protoargument-structure which is a structured representation of arguments based on thematic hierarchy:

(Agent (Experiencer(Goal/Source/Location(Theme)))))

The hierarchy expresses which argument has more chance of getting into the subject position. If the predicate assigns an Agent thematic role, this argument must be mapped into the syntactic function of subject. If there is no Agent or Experience argument in the thematic grid of the verb, the less prominent Goal/Source or Theme argument can get into the subject position.

As we described above, our agrammatic patients often gave answers in which they listed argument Ns or DPs (Type A and argument enumeration part of Type B answers). During the analysis of these kinds of answers, we found that the argument assignment was not random. The selection of arguments was connected with their **position in the thematic hierarchy and the 'animacy' semantic feature**, consequently the argument activation depended on the type of target verb.

Table 8.5 shows the distribution of arguments produced first in the different verb subgroups. (The numbers in parentheses show the number of total occurrences of a given argument: number of occurrences of an argument produced first linearly in the list plus the number of the same argument appearing as second or third element in another argument list.)

Based on the distribution of arguments the following thematic role preference was found in the different predicate types:

Transitive verbs   **Agent > Theme**
(*[+animate] object constituent*)
Transitive verbs   **Theme > Agent**
(*[–animate] object constituent*)
Two-place verbs   **Goal > Agent**
(*locative constituent*)
Three-place verbs   **Theme > Agent > Goal**
(*object+locative constituent*)
Three-place verbs   **Theme > Goal/Benefactive > Agent**
(*object+dative constituent*)

The subjects were able to produce every type of argument (Agent, Theme, Goal, Benefactive) but a difference was found in the distribution of arguments activated first.

Table 8.5. Distribution of arguments activated first (the total number of activated arguments including first activated is indicated in parentheses)

Type of verb	Agent	Goal/ Benefactive	Goal/ Source	Theme
Two-place [+anim.]	12 (13)	–	–	6 (12)
Two-place [-anim.]	10 (18)	–	–	52 (60)
Two-place [locative]	7 (8)	–	11 (13)	–
Three-place [locative]	10 (11)	–	5 (10)	16 (26)
Three-place [dative]	0 (5)	4 (6)	–	10 (13)

Activation of the arguments lower in the thematic hierarchy was more frequent than more prominent arguments of a given predicate (e.g. Theme > Benefactive > Agent; Theme > Agent; Goal > Agent). Two exceptions were found: the Agent > Goal order in the 'three-place locative' group and the Agent > Theme order in the 'transitive [+animate]' group. Comparing the proportions of arguments, a **remarkable contrast** was found between the activation of **Agent** and **Theme** arguments in the 'transitive [–animate]' and 'three-place dative' verb groups. In the case of the 'three-place locative' group the Agent ><Theme contrast was not so sharp, rather, the Goal/Source><Theme and the Agent ><Goal/Source contrasts were considerable. The contrast was also less sharp between the Agent and Goal arguments in the 'two-place locative' type of verbs.

The data show that the **less prominent Theme argument was activated faster** than the other arguments if the predicate assigned the thematic role of Theme mapped to an object NP specified as [–animate]. Activation of the Theme argument fell behind the Agent only if the verb was reversible (if the Theme thematic role was mapped into an object specified as [+animate, +human]).

Considering the total numbers of activated arguments, only the 'Theme [-animate] >< other arguments' contrast remained, the contrasts among the other arguments had been equalized. The Agent ><Theme [+animate] contrast also 'disappeared' when considering the total number of arguments.

The **Theme [–animate] argument** seems to be a preferred argument. Among the elements of the subcategorization list, mostly the Theme thematic role was assigned first. The verb–Theme argument relationship seems to be closer than the verb–other argument connection.

Case assignment in isolated arguments

The argument Ns and DPs were mostly produced without a case marker but case marked forms also occurred. Proportions of case marked forms in 'isolated argument assignment' answers were slight compared to the caseless forms. [Theme argument N with accusative: (4.5); Goal argument N with locative case marker: (13.0); Benefactive argument with dative case marker: (16.6). Case marker substitutions: Theme argument: (4.5); Agent argument: (3.6); Goal arguments: (8.6); Benefactive argument: (0.]

According to GB Case Theory case can be assigned under Government. The verb governs its complements and assigns them abstract cases. Hungarian has a morphologically rich case system; cases are realized morphologically and marked by overt case markers (only the nominative case is marked by a 'zero' morpheme). The verb idiosyncratically assigns case endings to their arguments, this information is indicated in the subcategorization frame (as a case frame). Case assignment can be realized in two ways:

1. If we assume that root-form argument Ns are inserted into the base structure, further morphological operations are needed to produce the appropriate case marked forms according to the information specified in the subcategorization list. This process assumes intact lexical selection of the given case marker from the 'grammatical marker lexicon' and intact morphosyntactic procedures that assign the overt case markers to the argument nouns.
2. We can also assume that the lexical entry of the noun involves the root form and all inflected variants of the noun. In this case, complete case marked forms can be retrieved from the lexicon and inserted into given syntactic slots. The verb assigns the case by checking the case markers of the NPs in the argument positions.

Both procedures seem to be possible on the cognitive level and are supported by processing data. The latter solution would correspond to a non-compositional holistic access regarding morphology combined with a decompositional secondary checking.

The aphasic subjects' performance indicates that the root forms (nominative) are generally accessible, our aphasic subjects rarely used a case marked form or direct holistic lexical access in their isolated argument answers. The tendency to omit case markers indicates a dysfunction of the syntactic structure building operations that can not create the minimally required syntactic domain (VP) needed in the case-assignment procedure. The slot of the case assigner (V) and the slot of the case marked constituent (N or N + I) are not available at the same time, only one nominal category slot is delivered and filled in by a lexical element.

The clausal answers (Types B and C)

After the activation of the available information from the lexical entry of the verb (argument-structure and thematic information), the agrammatic patients tried to insert the activated arguments into syntactic structure. The syntactic structure building mechanisms however, were also disturbed, they generated **both well-formed** and **agrammatic** sentences. (These sentences involved target or paraphasia predicates.)

Table 8.6. Proportion of agrammatic and well-formed sentences

	II/A Two-place [+anim]	II/B Two-place [−anim]	II/C Two-place [loc.]	III/A Three-place [loc.]	III/B Three-place [dat.]
Agrammatic S	47.5	58.4	44.0	58.3	42.1
Well-formed S	52.5	41.5	56.0	41.6	57.8
Total	40	65	25	24	19

Some agrammatic sentences were **(a) incomplete clause**, e.g. VO*, SVO*, SLVO* etc., because the complement NPs were deleted or the previously retrieved arguments were lost again when the subjects wanted to frame them into the slots of the phrase structure (into the complement or subject/ Topic positions).[2] Other agrammatic sentences were due to **(b) deletion of formatives**. The complete phrase structure was not built because of the lack of formatives (closed class items): case markers, verb inflections (agreement of the verb inflectional ending with the definiteness or indefiniteness of the object) and determiners/articles were deleted. (See Appendices 8.2. and 8.3. for examples.)

Word order in the clausal answers

Our subjects produced different permutations of surface word orders in the clausal answers. In Hungarian the verb's arguments can be freely topicalized but the sentence is (more) unmarked if the Agent NP or a constituent specified for [+human] or [+animate] semantic feature is preposed to the topic position. Our aphasic patients proved to be very sensitive to these features and to the prominent relations in the argument hierarchy.

The word order variations in the different verb groups were the following [note: (1) the verbs in these sentences were target or paraphasia verbs!; (2) word orders with highest occurrence are indicated **by bold letters**; word orders that occurred only one or two times are indicated in parentheses]:

a. **'Transitive [+animate]'/ reversible**
   V > SV > VO*> *SVO*, VC, SOV* > (OV, SVC, CVS, VS, VS', SVO, SCV)
b. **'Transitive [–animate]'/irreversible**
   VO* > V > VO > *VS,VC, SVO** > (SV, SVO*, VOC*, OV, SOV, OSV, SVC, CVS)
c. **'Two-place verbs with locative complement'**
   V > SV > (VS, VO, LV, VL, SVL, VL*)
d. **'Three-place with locative complement'**
   V > *VO* > *VO**> (LVO, VOL*, VO*L*, SV, VDO*, LV, VSO*, CVS
e. **'Three-place verbs with dative complement'**
   V > *VO*, SDOV* > (DVO*, SOVD, VDO, DSVO*, VO, VC, VSO)

V, SV, VO (VO*) word orders were always higher than other word order variations, across all permutations produced by the patients.

When the predicate did not assign the Theme argument ('Two-place locative') or there was no animacy contrast between the Theme and Agent arguments, the number of **V** and **SV** structures was higher.

In the case of those predicates that required Theme arguments and in which an animacy contrast was found between the Agent and Theme arguments, the **V, VO, VO*** answers occurred in the highest proportion.

Generating the types (a–e) of sentences, the aphasics used three main principles:

1. *'Insert the [+animate] [+human] argument into the subject or Topic position'.*

In the transitive/reversible verb group the Theme argument was also specified as [+animate] [+human], giving the possibility of 'perspective reversing': the 'original' Theme argument was mapped into the subject position of a one-place verb as Agent. (Some SV answers belonged to this kind of sentence type in this verb group.)

2. *'Keep the predicate and the Theme argument together'.*

3. If other information is not available/*accessible 'try to build the most simple structure selecting a one-place predicate'.*

These 'tendencies' are parallel to the strategies used by the subjects on the semantic mapping level:

- the **Agent** argument was activated first in higher proportion in the case of the 'transitive/reversible' verb group;
- in the case of the other predicates the **Theme** arguments were activated first which can be connected to the strategy: among the elements of the subcategorization list, 'map first the less prominent

argument into the syntactic frame. Construct the [V+O complement] structure first.'

Summary

We investigated the ability of two Broca's aphasic patients to produce simple active sentences which involved verbs of different argument structures with varying morphological complexity.

'Task specificity', which is a characteristic feature of aphasic performance, appeared in our investigation as well. Although our Broca patients omitted main verbs from their spontaneous speech, omission of verbs was not characteristic of their performance in an 'action naming task' rather, substitution of verbs occurred. Our subjects could retrieve one- or two-place verbs (target and paraphasia predicates) in a relatively high number (mean score of total verb answers in different verb groups involving the substitutions): 54.8/ 'one-place'; 71.0/ 'two -place'; 66.6/ 'three-place'). The proportion of the target verbs was lower than the ratio of the substituted predicates in the two-, or three-place verb types, which showed a lexical selection disorder in verb retrieval.

We found that the representational complexity of the verbs had a direct effect on the accessibility of the predicates. The 'morphologically simple one-place predicates' were produced in the highest number. Much lower proportions were found in the 'morphologically complex one-place' predicates and in the transitive verbs, and only some verbs were activated in the three-place verb groups. Production of the directional motion verbs proved to be the most difficult for the patients. These data showed that the argument structure complexity of the verb is important but not the only factor in the lexical selection of predicates. The semantic representational and morphological complexity of the predicate is also relevant in the lexical-semantic selection of the verbs.

Although the phonological form of the target verb was often not accessible for the aphasics, they could retrieve other specific information represented in the lexical entry of the verb. Argument structure and thematic information were partly accessible. Activation of the arguments was not random but related to the thematic hierarchy. The less prominent arguments were produced faster. The Theme argument specified as [−animate] was always the most preferred argument in the semantic and syntactic mapping procedures.

When there was no animacy contrast between the Agent and Theme argument, more Agent arguments were produced first than Theme arguments. The data show that the subjects used three principles in the semantic and syntactic mapping processes:

1. Map the [+animate], [+human] argument into the subject or Topic position, treating it as an Agent.

2. Construct first the verb-object complement structure, map the less prominent Theme argument specified as [−animate] first into the object position of the syntactic frame.
3. Construct the most simple (S)V structure if more information is not available from the semantic representation of the verb, selecting a one-place predicate.

Dysfunction of the syntactic structure building mechanisms had a connection with the lexical accessibility of formatives and nominal elements of the phrase structure. The reduced capacity to preserve the previously activated argument Ns or NPs had a role in the unsuccessful structure building operations. The previously activated argument nouns were often not preserved – they were not inserted into the given positions of the constituent structure – during the selection of the phonetic form of the verb. This resulted in incomplete clauses or fragments. The formatives were also not obtainable, they were not assigned to the appropriate slots of the case frame. This also resulted in agrammatic sentences. The semantic and syntactic mechanisms rarely operated in a parallel way or in coordination. The number of well-formed or complete clauses was very low in the case of predicates which assigned more complex argument structure.

Based on the data, agrammatic performance can be interpreted by those asynchronic mechanisms that cannot function simultaneously on/between the level of semantic operations (activation of argument-structure and thematic information) and syntactic processing (procedures that construct the syntactic phrase structure and map the arguments/thematic roles into the syntactic frame).

Appendix 8.1: Examples for typical answers in Types A–C

A. Isolated argument(s)

1. target: A férfi virágot ad a nônek. – The man gives flowers to the women.

   Anyuka ... virág ... A virág ... Férje ....
   [mother-nom ... flower-nom ... the flower-nom ... husband-gen-2sg]

2. target: A nô kiveszi a levelet a levélszekrénybôl. – The woman takes the letter out from the pillar-box.

   Levél ... Levélszekrény... Szekrénybe....
   [letter-nom ... pillar-box-nom ... wardrobe-into]

3. target: A fiú meghámozza a banánt. – The boy peels the banana.

   Banánt ... A fiú... banánt ....
   [banana-acc ... the boy-nom ... banana-acc ...]

B. Argument assignment > verb selection/clausal answer

1. target: A fiú felszáll a buszra. – The boy gets on the bus.

   Busz ... Fiú majd jön.
   [bus-nom ... Boy later come-3sg]

2. target: A férfi beleteszi a paradicsomot a zacskóba. – The man puts the tomato into the small bag.

   Mi ez?... Ja, paradicsom ... Paradicsom ... Egy sok paradicsom ... Szatyor és zacskó és paradicsom ... Kéri...
   [What is it?... Ah, tomato-nom ...Tomato-nom ... One many tomato ... Bag-nom and small bag-nom and tomato-nom ... ask-3sg-def. for ...]

3. target: A fiú kiönti a narancslevet a pohárba. – The boy pours out the orange juice into the glass.

   fiú... A fiúnak ... Nem ... 'Dzsúsz' ... Önti ... Kiönti a 'dzsúszt' ... A pohárba kiönti a 'dzsúszt'.
   [The boy-nom ... The boy-dat ... No ... Juice-nom ... Pour-3sg-def ... Prefix:out-pour-3sg-def the juice-acc. ...The glass-into prefix:out-pour-3sg-def the juice-acc.]

C. Clausal answer

1. target: A fiú átmegy a zebrán. – The boy is crossing the street /zebra.

   Kimegy a zebrán.
   [prefix :out-go-3sg the zebra-on]

2. target: A fiú kiönti a narancslevet a pohárba. – The boy pours out the juice into the glass.

   Önteni. Önteni a limonádét.
   [Pour-infinit. Pour-infin. the lemonade-acc]

3. target: A lány felébreszti a fiút. – The girl wakes up the boy.

   Alszik ... Letakarja.
   [Sleep-3sg....Prefix-cover-3sg-def]

Appendix 8.2: Examples for agrammatic – incomplete sentences

1. target: A fiú feltörli a tejet. – The boy wipes up the milk.

   A tej ... tej ... és nem jó. Tej és ... letörölni.
   [The milk-nom ... milk-nom ... and it is not good. Milk-nom and ...wipe-infinitive]

2. target : A fiú lekapcsolja a villanyt. – The boy switches the light off.

   Villany és és rá... És fiú lekapcsolja.
   [Light-nom and and onto ... And boy-nom switch-3sg.def off.]

Appendix 8.3: Examples for deletion of formatives in agrammatic sentences

1. target: A férfi fölszeleteli az uborkát. – The man-nom slice-3sg.def. the cucumber-acc

   Uborka ... Szeletelni. Férfi föl ... szeleteli uborkát.
   [Cucumber-nom ... Slice-infin. Man-nom prefix ... slice-3sg.def. cucumber-acc.

2. target : A lány elülteti a virágot. – The girl-nom plant-3sg.def. the flower-acc

   Virág... Elültetni virágot.
   [Flower-nom ... Plant-infin. flower-acc]

3. target: A fiú beleteszi a kenyeret a pirítóba. – The boy-nom prefix-put-3sg.def. the (slice of) bread-acc the toaster-into.

   Kenyér..Szeletelni...Odaadni kenyér.
   [Bread-nom...Slice-infin...Prefix-give-infin bread-nom.]

Notes

[1.] The 'transitive' group involved verbs that took single direct object NPs; the 'alternative dative' verbs like send, allowed [_NP], [_NP NP] and [_NP PP] subcategorization alternations, and (x,y), (x,y,z) argument structure possibilities; the 'non-alternating dative' verbs like carry, allowed two subcategorization possibilities: [_NP] and [_NP PP], and two argument structure alternations: (x,y), (x,y,z) ; the 'two complement' group consisted of verbs that allowed two subcategorizations and two argument structures:

1. *accept*   [_NP   (x, y)
                 S^1]   (x, Proposition)

   Those verbs belonged to the 'four complement' group that allowed two subcategorizations and four argument structures (Grimshaw, 1979):

2. *remember*   [_NP   (x, y)
                 S^1]   (x, Proposition)
                          (x, Question)
                          (x, Interrogative)

[2.] The asterisk (*) marks the deletion of the given constituent, D:dative complement, L:locative complement, C:other complement, S^1: sentential complement.

Chapter 9
Moving verbs in agrammatic production

NA'AMA FRIEDMANN

Introduction

Broca's aphasics with agrammatism suffer from a severe deficit in their ability to handle verbs. Until the early 1980s, the accepted account was that verb inflections are omitted in agrammatism. This was probably due to the fact that in English, patients produce bare verbs. In 1984, Grodzinsky looked at cross-linguistic data, and showed that the appropriate description of the data is substitution rather than omission of inflections: in languages in which the bare verb is well formed, the inflection is substituted by a zero morpheme; in languages in which a bare verb is not an option, substitution with a different inflection occurs. This ends up in inflection omission in languages like English, and in inflection substitution in languages like Hebrew.

In this chapter cross-linguistic data will be further used to show that agrammatics know even better than that: not only do they know not to omit the inflection when inflection omission creates a non-word, but their substitutions are also very constrained, in a way that lends itself to a syntactic description.

The structure of the argument advocated in this chapter will be as follows. First, it will be shown from a study in Hebrew and Arabic that not all inflections (and therefore not all functional categories) are impaired in agrammatic production. Some, subject–verb agreement for example, are preserved. Then, cross-linguistic data will be presented to show that even in the impaired domains, the bare verb (zero inflection) is not always preferred over other forms. The claim will be that the preference is not for bare forms, but for non-finite forms. Then it will be shown from a study of 11 Hebrew-speaking agrammatics that the infinitive is not always the preferred form as well. The conclusion will be that verb forms are chosen according to their syntactic properties of movement within the syntactic tree.

Are all function words equally impaired?

When looking at the empirical evidence to examine the extent of function word impairment, it seems that not all of them are impaired in agrammatic production. Some non-lexical nodes are indeed impaired, yet nodes in other parts of the structure (the phrase marker) are spared. Several non-lexical elements have already been shown to be intact in agrammatic production: among them case (Menn and Obler, 1990 for Finnish and Polish), coordination conjunctions (Menn and Obler, 1990; Friedmann, 1998) and negation markers (Lonzi and Luzzatti, 1993).

Even in the domain of inflections, not all inflections are equally impaired. A study of 13 Hebrew and Palestinian Arabic speaking agrammatic patients used sentence repetition and inflection completion tasks to examine the production of verb inflections (Friedmann, 1998). When looking at the agrammatics' production in these tasks, a dissociation between tense and agreement is apparent: tense inflection is impaired (even in an easy task such as repetition of a simple four-word sentence), but subject–verb agreement is almost intact. The difference between tense and agreement is significant both for Hebrew repetition, $\chi^2 = 142.96$, p << 0.0001; for Hebrew completion, $\chi^2 = 258.38$, p << 0.0001; and for Arabic completion, $\chi^2 = 34.82$, p << 0.0001. Patients produced tense errors almost exclusively – they substituted tense inflection, but did not make agreement errors in agreement completion or in repetition tasks (Tables 9.1 and 9.2). Each individual patient tested has shown this pattern of results.

Table 9.1. Verb inflection production tasks in Hebrew (11 patients) % substitution errors (number of errors/total)

	Tense errors		Agreement errors	
Repetition	16%	(143/912)	0%	(4/912)
Completion	42%	(322/760)	4%	(24/596)

Table 9.2. Verb completion task in Palestinian Arabic (two patients) % substitution errors (number of errors/total)

	Tense errors		Agreement errors	
Completion	69%	(31/45)	9%	(4/46)

Studies in other languages point in the same direction. For example, De Bleser and Luzzatti (1994) have examined past-participle agreement in a structured production task, and found a considerable preservation of this agreement inflection. (Most of the tasks in non-embedded sentences were performed at around 90% correct for both patients.)

In Spanish, verb agreement was also found to be much better preserved than tense inflection: using a sentence completion procedure, Benedet, Christiansen and Goodglass (1998) found that their six Spanish-speaking agrammatics produced only 5.5% correct verbal tense, but produced 63.8% correct subject–verb agreement. In English they found a similar pattern of results for the seven agrammatics they examined, but with a smaller difference: the English-speaking agrammatics produced 42% correct agreement and around 15% correct tense.

The same was found in French: the agrammatic patient Mr Clermont, reported in Nespoulous, Dordain, Perron, Jarema and Chazal (1988, 1990), had only tense errors in spontaneous speech, but no verb agreement errors.

The finding of intact agreement again rebuts the claim that agrammatics do not have syntactic trees at all, or lack all functional categories (Goodglass and Mayer, 1958; Myerson and Goodglass, 1972; Caplan and Futter, 1986; Ouhalla, 1993). Without the lower part of the syntactic tree, a correct verb agreement would be impossible. This situation calls for a more refined structural description that enables a distinction between the spared and impaired elements.

What are the types of verb inflection errors across languages?

After delimitating the substitutions to a subpart of verb inflections, the next step is to specify the exact types of inflection substitutions that do occur across languages.

Studies of agrammatic production in various languages have reported that patients tend to fall back on certain verb forms and use them excessively and incorrectly. These forms exist in most of the reported languages, but, interestingly, they exhibit cross-linguistic variation: agrammatics in different languages use different replacing forms. Therefore, these phenomena have also received different accounts. (See Table 9.3 for the data and related accounts.)

The use of bare verbs in English

Errors like the use of the verb 'give' instead of 'gives' in sentences like the following (1) were first described as *omissions* of inflectional morphemes.

1. The boy *give* to the girl a cookie. (Mr Franklin, in Menn, 1990)

These omissions were mainly attributed to one of two factors:

(i) Phonological characteristics of the non-stressed morphemes: Kean (1977) for example, argued that phonological words are preserved in agrammatic output, whereas clitics are omitted.

(ii) Lexical access deficit: the 'closed class lexicon' was said to be impaired in agrammatism, and because inflections are part of this lexicon, they are impaired and omitted (Bradley, Garrett and Zurif, 1980).

Table 9.3. Verb forms used in different languages: data and related accounts

Data	Accounts
Use of bare verbs in English	⇒ Inflection omission a. Phonological impairment (Kean, 1977) b. Closed class impairment (Bradley, Garrett and Zurif, 1980)
	⇒ Inflection substitution Preferred substitution to zero morpheme (Grodzinsky,1984)
Use of gerunds in English and infinitives in German	⇒ Nominalization (Goodglass and Geschwind, 1976; Saffran, Schwartz and Marin, 1980)
Use of participles in Italian	⇒ Preference of less marked forms over marked forms (Lapointe, 1985)
Finite verb omission in spontaneous speech	⇒ 'Averbia' — verb retrieval deficit (Zingeser and Berndt, 1990)

The use of gerunds in English and infinitives in German

Another fact observed in the agrammatic verb production was that: in English, agrammatics also use the gerund form (-ing) rather frequently, and in German they use the infinitive (-en). An example in English is given in (2) and in German (3).

2. Baby, baby **crying** (R.H., in Goodglass, Gleason, Bernholtz and Hyde, 1972)
3. Drei Monate ich überhaupt nicht **reden** (Mr Meyer, in Stark and Dressler, 1990)

Because these are suffixed verb forms, this could not be explained by pure omission, and it was related to the idea that agrammatics use the verb to name an action. These forms were considered as *nominalizations* of the verb (Goodglass and Geschwind, 1976; Saffran, Schwartz and Marin, 1980).

The use of participles in Italian

Still, omission and nominalization do not cover the whole variety of overused verb forms. In Italian, patients also use the participle, as shown in (4) from Mr Verdi, in Miceli and Mazzucchi (1990).

4. Non c'é   il pollo   **mangiato**   il cane.
    Not there-is   the chicken   eat-participle   the dog.

In light of this (and other problems in the omission and nominalization descriptions) Lapointe (1985) and Lapointe and Dell (1989) argued that agrammatic aphasics have a problem accessing syntactic stores, and have fewer processing resources than normals, a fact which prevents them from accessing the more complex items in every verb-group. This, in turn, leads them to either replace the complex forms with morphosemantically less complex (less marked) forms, or to omit the verb altogether. The markedness metric is different for every language, and consequently, bare verbs and gerunds are used in English, but infinitives and participles are used in Italian.

Consideration of the accounts

The inflection omission account that claims that bare verbs are a result of omission of morphemes is both too strong and too weak. It is too strong, because it predicts all inflectional affixes to be omitted, contrary to fact. It can not explain why some inflectional suffixes (such as the German infinitival suffix -en, and the English progressive suffix -ing) are preserved, and even overused, whereas other suffixes (such as the English suffix -ed) are omitted.

The omission account is also too weak, because it fails to explain the difficulties agrammatics have with inflectional morphology in languages with non-concatenative morphology. Recall that the phonological account claimed that agrammatics simply omit clitics, because they are not stressed. If so, agrammatics in languages in which inflectional morphology constitutes part of the 'phonological word' are predicted to be lucky, and not to have trouble with inflections. Nevertheless, Grodzinsky (1984) brought evidence from several languages to show that even in these languages, agrammatics' ability to inflect is not spared. In Hebrew, for example, the errors are substitution rather than omission errors: agrammatics do provide inflections – only they are the wrong ones.

Grodzinsky (1984) therefore proposed a unified syntactic account for both omissions and substitutions. According to him, non-lexical terminals (namely, everything which is not a noun, a verb or an adjective) are deleted from the agrammatic representation. The inflectional errors result from the underspecification of inflectional terminals. In languages in which the verb is well formed without inflection, a bare verb (or a verb with zero inflection) is produced. In languages in which bare verbs are not well-formed words (when zero inflection is not an option), the inflection is randomly chosen, and a substitution occurs. Omissions, then, are substitutions with zero morpheme, and this is the preferred substitution. Later studies proved that indeed, cross-linguistically, this generalization holds: agrammatics do not omit inflections in a way that creates verb forms which are non-words in their languages (Menn and Obler, 1990; Mimouni and Jarema, 1997).

Although this zero-morpheme approach accounts for a much bigger part of the data, it has two major problems. First, it cannot account for the dissociation just sketched between tense and agreement, and for the other preserved non-lexical categories. Secondly, it cannot account for languages in which the bare verb (verb + zero inflection) is a well-formed existing word, yet agrammatics do not use it, or prefer a suffixed infinitive over it. Apparently this is the case in German, Dutch and Icelandic, where the bare verb is used in some singular imperatives and singular present tense forms, and the infinitive is suffixed.

The data show that although in German, for example, the stem is a well-formed word, it is not used. The ten German-speaking agrammatics reported in Kolk and Heeschen (1992) for instance, used the infinitive as main verbs in matrix clauses 53% of the time, but never used the stem incorrectly (0%), although the stem is an existing verb form.

In Dutch, Bastiaanse and Van Zonneveld (1998) report the use of both the stem and the infinitive, but the infinitive is preferred over the stem (13 substitutions by infinitives compared to eight by stems).

Similarly in Icelandic, the bare verb is well formed and the infinitive is inflected with the suffix -a. Nevertheless, Magnúsdóttir and Thráinsson's (1990) patient Togga did not omit verbal inflection: she either used the infinitive, or substituted the inflection.

So, the omission account does not work here, and neither does the later version of inflection substitution (Grodzinsky, 1984), because the bare form is not always the preferred form. Agrammatics do substitute and not omit, but it is not the case that they prefer the zero inflection. Sometimes (in English for example) they indeed prefer the bare forms, but for other reasons, as will be discussed shortly.

The *nominalization* account is unjustified, because there is no evidence for nominal properties of the verb forms used. In sentential contexts, the gerund and the infinitive appear in verb distribution and not in noun distribution: they never appear after determiners, with adjectives, as a complement of prepositions and non-copular verbs. They seem to preserve the predicate argument structure of the verb, appearing in NP V-ing NP constructions etc. (Lapointe, 1985).

As for the *morphosemantic account* (Lapointe, 1985), a morphological account that claims that agrammatics only substitute marked forms for less marked forms cannot handle the fact that the use of an infinitive instead of an inflected verb has implications for word order as will be shown below. Furthermore, the markedness scales succeed in many cases to describe the data, but because these scales are arbitrarily ordered, they offer a well-organized description rather than an explanation for the data. This chapter will try to show how verbal complexity ordering is derived in a non-arbitrary way from the syntactic properties of the phrase marker and the agrammatic deficit.

We are left with the following set of seemingly unrelated facts: use of the verb stem without the inflections, which counted as omission and afterwards as substitution for a zero-inflection; use of infinitives and gerund which counted as nominals, and participles which counted as 'less marked forms', and agrammatics who speak Dutch, German and Icelandic who prefer the suffixed infinitive over the well-formed stem. Is there a unified way to account for all these phenomena?

A unified account for the phenomena

I believe that the key to understanding these phenomena lies in the idea that incorrect verb forms are non-finite, replacing finite, fully inflected ones. What makes infinitives, gerunds and participles a group is their non-finiteness.[1]

So in English, inflections are not omitted, neither are they replaced by zero inflection. The English inflected verbs are simply replaced by infinitives. This is also why in German, Dutch and Icelandic agrammatics do not use the (finite) stem: they prefer to use the non-finite forms – the infinitive and the participle.

The use of non-finite forms derives from the structure of the pruned agrammatic phrase marker and results from the fact that some of the functional categories are not projected in the tree. The idea is that the replacing forms are verb forms which do not have to move to pruned nodes in the tree, and that they replace verb forms that need these nodes in order to be licensed. Before going into the exact mechanism of verb inflection in agrammatic production, a brief summary of the relation between verb inflection and nodes in the syntactic tree is given. Then the Tree Pruning Hypothesis of agrammatic production will be presented to explain the use of non-finite forms in agrammatism.

Syntactic tree pruning and verb inflection deficit

Verb movement and inflection

According to current linguistic theories, the verb is inserted from the lexicon into V^0 in the VP, then raises to the Agreement node in order to collect its agreement inflection, and then to the Tense node in order to collect its tense inflection (Pollock, 1989, 1994) see Figure 9.1.

A checking account such as Chomsky's 1993 minimalist program also claims that verbs raise from VP to the functional categories T and AGR, but with a different motivation: verbs move in the tree in order to *check* their inflectional features, rather than to collect them.

The exact movement pattern of a verb depends on two factors: the language and the verb form. An inflected verb usually moves high in the tree, whereas a non-finite bare verb does not have to move, and stays in a low node, sometimes even inside the VP. Non-finite verbs differ with respect to the number of functional nodes they require and the height of their movement target.

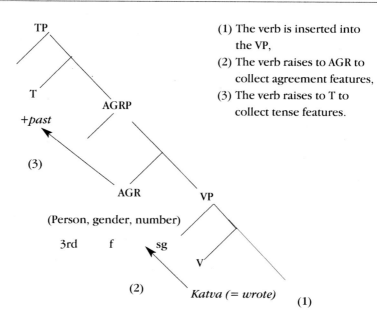

(1) The verb is inserted into the VP,

(2) The verb raises to AGR to collect agreement features,

(3) The verb raises to T to collect tense features.

Figure 9.1. An example of a Hebrew verb moving to AGR and T to collect (or check) its inflectional features. 'katva' = write-third-person, singular, feminine, past. (Partial syntactic tree)

The Tree Pruning Hypothesis

According to the Tree Pruning Hypothesis (TPH, Friedmann, 1994; Friedmann and Grodzinsky, 1997), the agrammatic tree is pruned from the Tense node and up (see Figure 9.2). The Tense node and the nodes above it are inaccessible to the agrammatic speaker. This induces a variety of deficits in the agrammatic speech: a deficit in tense inflection (but not in agreement which is below the pruning site), and deficits in *Wh* question and embedding production (Friedmann, 1998). Because inflected verbs in many languages have to move up in the tree in order to collect (or check) their inflection, a pruned tree means that verbs cannot move all the way up to get checked. Therefore, only verbs that do not need to raise higher than the pruning site are correctly produced.

So which verb forms will be produced in agrammatic speech?

Because the tree is pruned, movement to the high branches is hampered. If movement is prevented, verbs can not move to collect their inflections. Thus the aphasic can only produce the verb as it is, without movement. The verb forms that do not move are exactly the forms that in many languages do not have to collect inflections – the non-finite forms.

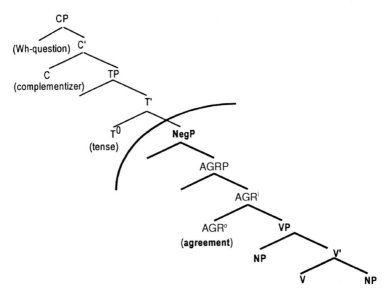

Figure 9.2. Agrammatic pruned tree (Tree Pruning Hypothesis, Friedmann and Grodzinsky, 1997).

Forms which can be licensed without movement to pruned nodes will be correctly produced, and will not suffer from pruning of functional categories. Contrariwise, forms which are not licensed in a low node, and have to move to pruned nodes in order to be licensed, can not be correctly produced. The forms that would appear instead of them would be forms that can be licensed in a lower node, that is, non-finite forms. Consequently, inflected verbs are replaced by infinitives, participles or gerunds.

Take for example the German verb 'gehen' (= go): if the sentence required the infinitive form *gehen*, which stays down in the VP, it would be produced appropriately as *gehen*. On the other hand, if the sentence required the inflected *geht*, or *ging* (= goes, went), the verb would not be able to move to T (Tense node) and C for tense collecting/checking, and it would therefore appear in the infinitive form *gehen* instead of the inflected form.[2]

Agrammatics will only use forms which are licensed in nodes lower than the impaired node. These forms are in many languages the gerund, the infinitive and the participle. And indeed, these forms are the verb forms agrammatics use across languages, instead of the higher aiming inflected forms.

Thus, the tree pruning is the crucial factor here: as long as verbs move below the pruning site, no problem is expected. But when a verb needs to move to nodes in the pruned zone, then the inflection deficit arises. As a result, in each language, agrammatics use verb forms that do not have to raise higher than the pruning site in their language, instead of inflected verbs that need to move higher than the pruning site.

The relation between verb form and word order

If the overuse of non-finite verbs should really be accounted for by a pruned tree which prevents long verb-movement, this should have implications for word order. I argued that a verb is produced in its non-finite form because it does not have finite functional categories to move to. An immediate prediction of this claim is that when the verb is non-finite it should also appear in a low node, that is, in the place which is preserved for non-finite verbs. On the other hand, if, as other accounts for the preponderance of infinitives in agrammatism suggested, agrammatics produce an infinitive instead of a finite verb because it is morphosemantically simpler, it should not affect word order, and non-finite forms should appear in the finite verb position.

In order to test the contrasting predictions, we should look at languages in which the finite and non-finite verbs appear in different structural positions. We should also choose languages in which the position of the infinitive and the finite verbs is discernible from the produced sentence.

In these languages, we shall then look at the position of the infinitive which is produced instead of the inflected verb. If the infinitive is produced in the same place as the finite – early in the sentence – it will support the morphological accounts. If, on the other hand, it appears at the infinitival position down the tree (namely, later in the sentence), it will support our claim that the verb has not moved up in the tree.

Lonzi and Luzzatti (1993) examined verb position in Romance languages such as Italian and French. They have shown that agrammatic aphasics produce finite and non-finite verbs in their correct positions. In Italian, finite verbs occur only before the adverb, and non-finites (infinitives and participles) appear both before and after the adverb. Lonzi and Luzzatti found that in spontaneous speech patients always obeyed this word order: in 41 out of 42 sentences, they put the verb in the correct position relative to the specifier-adverb, namely, they only once placed the finite verb incorrectly after the adverb. (No data is given as to the number of finite and non-finite verbs in the corpus analysed.)[3]

In French, finite verbs precede the negative particle *pas*, and infinitives follow it. Again, analysing spontaneous speech, Lonzi and Luzzatti found that when agrammatics produce the infinitive, they always produce it after the negation, and when a finite verb is produced, it appears before the negation.

Note, that this study included mainly correctly produced infinitives and not only infinitives replacing the finite verbs: both the French and the Italian speaking agrammatics in the corpus analysed from Menn and Obler (1990), for example, preferred to replace the inflected verbs with the participle rather than the infinitive. The two French agrammatics used only two infinitives out of 220 verbs, and the two Italian patients produced only four out of 175 verbs.

But the point remains the same: when a verb is produced correctly inflected, it has moved up and therefore it appears before the adverb. When it appears in the infinitive, both when the infinitive is required and when an inflected verb is required, it appears in the infinitival position.

Another critical case where the relation between verb inflection and verb position can be examined empirically is verb second Germanic languages. In many Germanic languages (such as Dutch, German, Icelandic and Scandinavian languages), the finite verb moves to the second position of the clause, after the first constituent – be it the subject, as in (5) or any other constituent as in (6).

S V O

5. de jongen   **loopt**   op straat
   the boy   walks   on street

XP V S O

6. langzaam   **loopt**   de jongen op straat
   slowly   walks   the boy on street

Whereas finite verbs move to second position, non-finite verbs (participles and infinitives), do not move and stay in final position, as seen in the sentences for German (7) and Dutch (8):[4]

7. a. V_{fin} 2nd: Konrad **schaute** aus   dem Fenster.
                         Konrad looked   out   of the window
   b. V_{inf} final: Konrad will   aus   dem Fenster **schauen**.
                         Konrad wants out of the window look-inf

8. a. V_{fin} 2nd: De boer   **melkt** de koe
                         the farmer milks   the cow
   b. V_{inf} final: De boer   wil   de koe **melken**
                         the farmer wants the cow milk-inf

V2 is a movement from V^0 to C^0 (through I^0). This is the reason for the difference in V2 languages between matrix and embedded clauses with respect to verb position: in embedded sentences the C node is already occupied by a complementizer, and therefore the verb cannot raise to C, and stays down in final position, as seen in sentence (9) in German. This is one of the most illustrative examples of the close connection between functional categories, head movement and verbal inflection.

9. Es ist kein Wunder, **dass** sich   Onkel Ringelhuth über nichts **wunderte**.
   It is no wonder,   **that** himself uncle Ringelhuth over nothing
                                                                wondered.

Consider how this might serve as one of the crucial tests for evaluating the accounts of infinitive use in agrammatism: a tree pruning account which entails no verb movement to T (and therefore also no subsequent movement to C) predicts that in V2 languages, the infinitive will not appear in second position but *in final position*. That is – whenever a verb appears in its non-finite form, and crucially, also when it appears inappropriately non-finite instead of finite, it should appear in the structural location of the non-finite forms – namely in its base-generated node (or after short movement to AGR to check Agreement features) at the end of the sentence. On the other hand, no consequence for word order derives from non-structural accounts: accounts of 'morphological' inflectional deficit predict a use of 'least effort' or 'default' form *in the same sentential position* of the required finite verb.

Data from structured tests and spontaneous speech in Germanic V2 languages verify the TPH prediction: when an infinitive is used even instead of a finite verb in matrix clause, it is almost always in final position. This has been found for Dutch and German, and some indications for verb position implication were also found for Swedish and Icelandic.

A study recently conducted by Bastiaanse and Van Zonneveld (1998) examined the question of the relation between finiteness and verb position. In this study, ten Broca's aphasics were required to complete sentences with a verb missing either in second or in final position, in matrix or embedded clause.

The results show that agrammatics have a hard time producing verbs in the moved position (second position), but they do not have problems producing verbs in their base-generated position, at the end of the sentence (see Table 9.4).

Table 9.4. The relation between verb position and verb production in Dutch: correct verb produced/total verbs produced

+fin V2 (matrix)	– fin final (matrix)	+fin final (embedded)	– fin final (embedded)
24/41	60/60	50/58	50/51

Source: Bastiaanse and Van Zonneveld (1998).

The difference between finite and non-finite verbs was striking: There was only one error out of 111 verbs in final position – in which a finite (past participle) was produced instead of an infinitive. Verbs in second position, on the other hand, were much harder to retrieve than verbs in final position, and were frequently substituted by non-finite forms. This tells us that agrammatics have difficulties in producing inflected verbs in second position, presumably because they cannot raise the verb to this position, and that the pattern of verb inflection is closely connected to the pattern of verb movement. Recall that the patients were only asked to produce a single verb in the required position and not the whole sentence. Thus, the incorrect use of non-finites also in second position should not be taken as an indication for the use of non-finite verbs in high nodes: the verbs were wrongly inflected because the patients were agrammatic aphasics who encounter a deficit of verb raising and inflection, and they therefore produced non-inflected verbs when required to produce a finite verb. Presumably, the verbs that appeared uninflected when required in second position would have appeared in final position in spontaneous speech.

This conjecture is borne out by data from spontaneous speech in Dutch and German: Kolk and Heeschen (1992) report use of infinitives in matrix clause in their ten German and eight Dutch patients' spontaneous speech. Their data again indicate exactly the result expected by a syntactic account: as seen in Table 9.5, almost all the inflected main verbs were produced in second position, which means that they moved to collect (or check) their inflection. Furthermore, when infinitives were produced as main verbs without an auxiliary (this analysis included only substituting infinitives [Kolk, personal communication, July 1997]), they appeared in sentence final position, the position of verbs that have not moved up the tree.

Table 9.5. Verb inflection and position in Dutch and German % correct (number of sentences/total)

	Infinitive in final position	Finite verb in second position
Dutch (8 patients, 139 sentences)	93% (64/69)	99% (69/70)
German (10 patients, 175 sentences)	86% (59/69)	97% (103/106)
Mean	**89% (123/138)**	**98% (172/176)**

Source: Kolk and Heeschen (1992), data processed from Table 5, p. 111.

Similar results have been reported for Dutch by Bastiaanse and Van Zonneveld (1998): in their three Dutch-speaking agrammatics' spontaneous speech, 45 out of 45 finite verbs were produced in second position, and 45 out of the 46 non-finites appeared in final position (note, also, the high rate of non-finites in agrammatic speech: half of the verbs!).

It might be that the inaccessibility of high nodes to verb movement is also the cause for word order deficit with regard to verb position noticed in SVO V2 languages such as Swedish and Icelandic.[5] Ahlsén and Darvins (1990) provide the spontaneous speech of a Swedish-speaking patient (Ms Garbo) who exhibits problems with tense inflection resulting both in finite tense substitutions and in infinitive for finite substitutions. This patient also produces matrix sentences with wrong verb position: although the order SVO is kept in sentences beginning with the subject, the patient produces sequences of the type Adverb–Subject–Verb (see (10)), instead of the required Adv–V–S order with the verb in second position.

10. Sen   han titta
    Then he   go-inf/part

The same phenomenon was also observed by Magnúsdóttir and Thráinsson (1990) for the Icelandic patient Togga:

11. Svo   hann sofna   i aftur
    Then he   fell asleep again

The word-order deficit in these two language may be the result of obstructed verb movement to C. Because CP is not available, the sentential adverb cannot settle in spec-CP and therefore it does not attract the verb to C^0. As a result, the verb stays low, and is produced after the subject even when there are other constituents in first position.[6] In Ms Garbo's speech, out of 16 verbs that appeared in non-second position in matrix clauses, 11 were infinitives.[7]

The relation between verb inflection and verb movement in agrammatism in these Scandinavian SVO V2 languages is still not sufficiently clear, and structured production tests are required to determine whether verb movement deficit is indeed correlated to the inflectional deficit. Compared to Dutch and German, it is more difficult to determine whether the verb has moved to C or not in these languages,[8] and the position of the non-finite verb relative to negation and sentential adverbs may come to our rescue and supply the answer. In these languages, moved verbs precede sentential adverbs and negation markers, whereas verbs that have not moved follow them. It is thus possible to enquire whether non-finite matrix verbs do not move high in the tree by eliciting sentences with adverbs or negations.

To conclude, V2 languages provide substantial evidence in favour of a syntactic account to non-finite verb use in agrammatism, and rule out lexical or morphological accounts for this phenomenon. Data from both structured tests and spontaneous speech analysis indicate that whenever a main verb appears in a non-finite form, it is also located down the tree, where non-finites live.

Note that infinitival verbs appear here in final position just as they would have appeared with auxiliary or modal in second position, but auxiliary/modal omission cannot be the right account for the abundance of infinitives, or for the infinitival final position. As Kolk and Heeschen (1992) rightfully note, normals use aux + infinitive constructions in only

10–14% of the sentences, and there is no reason to believe that agrammatics would prefer to use auxiliary constructions in 53% of the sentences, and then omit the auxiliary. True, agrammatics do use forms that usually require an auxiliary verb, but only because the forms they use are forms that do not carry tense, and therefore in normal syntax require an auxiliary to carry the inflection.

Verb omission: averbia or inflectional deficit?

Agrammatics frequently omit verbs in spontaneous speech and in picture description. This led researchers to claim that agrammatics have an additional problem: averbia (see for example Zingeser and Berndt, 1990). That is – in addition to their other deficits, they also have a special problem in the lexicon that prevents them from retrieving verbs.

In the Bastiaanse and Van Zonneveld (1998) study, Dutch-speaking agrammatics had 'verb retrieval' deficits in second position only (where the verb has to be inflected) but not in sentence final position (where it appears in a low node). This finding cannot be explained by lexical retrieval deficit. It indicates, rather, the strong relation between verb production and its sentential position, and raises the possibility that agrammatics omit verbs not due to a lexical retrieval deficit, but due to their inability to move them to the relevant functional categories in the syntactic tree and to inflect them correctly.

Another corroboration for this claim comes from a tense treatment study: Weinrich, Shelton, Cox and McCall (1997) report that their patients had severe tense-inflection deficit before treatment: they inflected only 5% and 17%, 22% of their verbs correctly for tense. At that stage, their patient also had verb-retrieval deficit: they produced only 36%, 43% and 53% of the required verbs. After treatment of tense production, when their tense inflection has improved significantly (to 92, 64 and 73% correct), their verb retrieval ability had strikingly doubled (to 89, 85 and 83%). This again suggests the involvement of inflection in verb production.

This poses a new type of explanation for verb omission in terms of verb movement. When agrammatics have to inflect a verb and move it to a pruned position, they sometimes prefer not to produce the verb at all. The deficit, then, is not a purely lexical deficit in the 'verb lexicon'. It is modulated, rather, by syntactic structure, and can be explained within the framework of pruned trees and the resulting verb movement deficit.

Thus, verb omissions may result from the same deficit that causes verb inflection errors: a syntactic deficit.

Infinitives in Hebrew

One of the important properties of the infinitives that are used in agrammatic production instead of inflected verbs is that they are *bare infini-*

tives: namely, they do not contain the 'to' morpheme. Agrammatics produce sentences of the form, but do not produce sentences like (13).

12. Dori drive a Porsche
     Dori to drive a Porsche

It is now clear why aphasics use verbs without the 'to' morpheme (see, for example, 'to' omissions in English and Dutch in Menn and Obler, 1990): 'to' is a tense morpheme, and is located in Tense node which is located in the pruned part of the tree. Whereas bare infinitives are licensed in low nodes, their inflection 'to' is not.

Consider the implications this has for the choice of replacing forms in a language that does not have a bare verb, and where its infinitive includes the 'to' as a bound inflection. In such a language, the infinitive also has to move up to tense node to collect (or check) its inflection. In this case, infinitives are expected not to be produced instead of finite verbs.

Fortunately we can test this in Hebrew, seeing as Hebrew is a language in which the infinitive is not bare. The Hebrew infinitive contains a morpheme which is the analogue of 'to' (the prefix 'le-'), and it is therefore parallel to the whole phrase 'to go' in English, and not only to the bare verb 'go'. Therefore, the infinitive in Hebrew must raise high like an inflected verb, to check its inflection. Another demonstration for the difference between the Hebrew infinitive and the English infinitive is the fact that the Hebrew infinitive does not appear as a complement of auxiliary verbs. Because it is inflected and occupies the Tense node, there is no place or need for an auxiliary. Furthermore, the movement pattern of the infinitive in Hebrew is just the same as the movement of the finite verb: arguments from word order of adverbs and infinitives show that they raise to the same high node in the syntactic tree as finites (Shlonsky, 1997).

The prediction, then, is that in Hebrew, unlike in German and Dutch, for example, infinitives will not be overused in agrammatic production. This prediction was tested in 11 Hebrew-speaking agrammatic patients (Friedmann, 1998).

Sentence repetition and verb completion in sentential context were used to assess inflection abilities and to find out whether agrammatic aphasics use infinitives instead of finite verbs in Hebrew. Errors were analysed in order to determine whether agrammatics substituted the infinitive for finite verbs, or kept all verb inflection errors within the finite paradigm.

The results were clear-cut: substitution errors were almost always within the finite paradigm (or possibly included substitution of the participle which is identical to the present tense). Errors were substitution of one tense for another, but almost never substitution of infinitival form for the finite.[9] Again, each individual patient showed the same pattern of results. The results for verb repetition and completion are presented in Table 9.6. The difference between finite infinitival substitutions is significant both for repetition: $\chi^2 = 148.95$, p << 0.0001, and for completion: $\chi^2 = 471.70$ p << 0.0001.

Table 9.6. Verb inflection production tasks in Hebrew (11 patients): comparing substitution errors of infinitives and wrongly inflected finites for a finite verb

| | Finite verb for finite verb (Tense substitution) | | Infinitive for finite verb | |
	% errors	(errors/total)	% errors	(errors/total)
Repetition	16%	(143/912)	0%	(2/912)
Completion	42%	(322/760)	2%	(16/1021)

The results show that all the Hebrew-speaking patients keep the distinction between finite and non-finite forms. They have a clear boundary between the two, and they do not cross it when substituting. The reason, we suggest, is that unlike in Germanic languages, the Hebrew infinitive also has to raise high in the tree, and therefore there is no use for it instead of other forms that have to raise . The conclusion is that the preference of agrammatics is not always for the infinitive, but rather for forms that do not have to raise high in the syntactic tree.

It seems, then, that the choice between the non-finite forms is dictated by the nature of their movement in each particular language: if the infinitive has to raise but the participle stays low, the participle will be the preferred form in this particular language. When the infinitive is not an option, tense substitutions will occur within the finite paradigm.

Summary

Although agrammatic production is usually described as impaired in all aspects of grammar and in all types of inflections, structured tests have shown that not all the inflections are equally impaired in agrammatic production. A study of 13 Hebrew- and Arabic-speaking agrammatics has shown that although tense inflection is severely impaired, agreement is unimpaired.

Therefore, a Tree Pruning Hypothesis was proposed (Friedmann and Grodzinsky, 1997), according to which the agrammatic phrase marker is pruned from the Tense node and up, thus impairing tense inflection and subordination, but leaving agreement inflection intact.

The main claim here is that the Tree Pruning Hypothesis is able to account for an additional phenomenon in agrammatic production: the overuse of some verb forms in various languages instead of inflected verbs, such as the bare verb in English, the infinitive in German and the participle in Italian.

Until now, the use of different verb forms in agrammatism has received different explanations. Here we suggested that the verb forms that are substituting for other forms are always forms that do not have to raise to pruned nodes of the syntactic tree in order to be licensed. Because non-finite forms – the infinitive, the participle and the gerund are in many languages the forms that do not move high in the tree, these are the forms that are abundant in agrammatic speech.

As a result, verb form substitution is tightly related to word order: in Germanic V2 languages such as Dutch and German, whenever an infinitive is used instead of an inflected verb, it also appears in a position within the low part of the tree, in final position, where verbs that did not move reside.

In addition, it has been shown that in Hebrew, where the infinitive has to move high in the tree, agrammatics do not use the infinitive instead of the finite verb. They only substitute within the finite paradigm, and they keep the finiteness distinction. This means that there is no general preference for the infinitive, but only when the infinitive does not have to move to high nodes of the phrase marker. This induces the diversity between substituting forms in different languages: in languages like Dutch and German, where the verb can stay down, it is produced as an infinitive. But in languages like Hebrew, where it does not have this option, a random tense is chosen.

In order to test this claim further empirically, more structured tests should be undertaken in languages with different patterns of verb movement. These tests should enable us to determine the target verb form, and the verb position within the tree, which can be established based on the relative order of the substituting form and clitics, adverbs and negation markers.

Notes

[1] In this respect, this claim is reminiscent of the conceptual move made by Wexler (1994) for children's use of infinitives, but with a different underlying cause: it is not the case that agrammatics think that tense is optional. Tense is defected and inaccessible to them, and so is the rest of the tree above it. Also in contrast to children, agrammatics make tense substitutions, which children never make.

[2] When it is a language in which this is not possible, namely, in case all verb forms have to raise to higher nodes, it is not directly predicted what would be produced in this case: the options are non-licensed, random form [to avoid phonological well-formedness violations (Grodzinsky, 1990)] a nominalization of the verb, or verb omission.

[3] Correct verb–adverb order was also found in a card-ordering task, but it is unclear whether this type of task is a pure production task or whether it involves grammaticality judgment, especially given that the patients decided on the final correct ordering after the experimenter had read the sequence to them.

[4] As Zwart (1993) notes, this final position may be followed by complement clauses and adjuncts.

[5] In Swedish only Ms Garbo's data was analysed, and in Icelandic only Togga's data, as

the two other cases were mildly impaired: the Swedish-speaking Mr Bergman had only three word order errors with respect to verb position, and the Icelandic-speaking Kiddi was very mildly impaired with an exceptionally low rate of errors in all measures, and therefore was not very informative for agrammatic production analysis.

6. The relative order of the subject and the verb is kept either because they both stay in VP or because both undergo short movement to a low maximal projection within the intact part of the tree – the subject to the specifier of the functional category, and the verb to its head.

7. A similar word order deficit with adjuncts in first position was also described by Hackl (1995) for German.

8. In SOV V2 languages such as German and Dutch there is abundant indication as to whether or not verb movement to second position has taken place, because their I and V are both final and therefore any content of VP makes it possible to judge whether the erroneously produced non-finite verb has moved to a finite position. Things are more complicated with SVO V2 languages, such as Scandinavian languages. Scandinavian languages (Swedish, Norwegian and Danish but not Icelandic) do not allow V-to-I movement, due to their poor inflectional paradigm. Yet, they do contain V-to-I-to-C movement.

9. Interestingly, this was also found for Hebrew-speaking normal children and SLI children: they do not use infinitives instead of finite verbs even in stages where their English-, French-, Dutch- and German-speaking counterparts do. (See Dromi, Leonard and Shteiman, 1993, for SLI children; Armon-Lotem, 1996; Berman and Armon-Lotem, 1996, for normal children.)

The preparation of this chapter was supported by a grant from the Israel Foundation Trustees.

Chapter 10
Verb retrieval, verb inflection and negation in agrammatic aphasia

ROELIEN BASTIAANSE, JUDITH RISPENS AND RON VAN ZONNEVELD

Introduction

Agrammatic aphasics have problems with the production of verbs. Several studies show that action naming is more impaired than object naming (e.g. Kohn, Lorch and Pearson, 1989; Zingeser and Berndt, 1990; Jonkers and Bastiaanse, 1996) and analysis of spontaneous speech demonstrates that the number of verbs is reduced. If verbs are produced, they often lack inflection (Saffran, Berndt and Schwartz, 1989; Thompson, Shapiro, Li and Schendel, 1995; Bastiaanse, Jonkers and Moltmaker-Osinga, 1995). It has been suggested that there is a relation between these two different tasks (e.g. Berndt, Michum, Haendiges and Sandson, 1997b), but this has never been numerically supported. It is not at all clear how the performance on an action naming test should relate to verb use in spontaneous speech. A low score on a test may reflect poor lexical retrieval, but there is no reason to assume *a priori* that this has direct consequences for the use of verbs in spontaneous speech. Many factors may facilitate or complicate verb production in spontaneous speech. A syntactic frame may help to access verbs, for example, whereas the necessity to inflect the verb or to produce the accompanying arguments may reduce verb retrieval. Apart from these linguistic factors, strategic aspects may play a role. Spontaneous speech offers the possibility to produce alternatives if the target verb cannot be found, but producing discourse may be more demanding, because no pictures, nor any other cues are present to give some guidance for word retrieval.

Accepting that the main problem of agrammatic aphasics is their grammatical deficit, the present experiments investigate how this relates to verb production in spontaneous speech. In the first part, the relation between action naming and the production of verbs in spontaneous speech will be addressed; the second experiment fractionates the verb production problem further, by distinguishing the morphological and syntactic aspects of inflection. It will be suggested that the underlying deficit causing verb retrieval problems in spontaneous speech is syntactic rather than lexical or morphological in nature. The last experiment focuses on an issue that is closely related to verb production in some languages but not in others, that is, the syntax of negation.

Action naming vs. spontaneous speech

In the first study, action-to-picture naming has been compared with lexical, morphosyntactic and argument structural aspects of the verb production in spontaneous speech.

Methods

Subjects

Eight agrammatic aphasics and eight normal controls participated in this study. The agrammatics were aphasic due to a single stroke. They were selected from a larger group of agrammatics by the criterion that they had produced at least 300 words spontaneous speech, the minimum amount that should be used for a spontaneous speech analysis (see e.g. Vermeulen, Bastiaanse and Van Wageningen, 1989; Brookshire and Nicholas, 1994). Only 'classic' agrammatics were included, meaning that telegraphic speech was a condition and that comprehension in a conversation was good. The relevant patient data are given in Table 10.1. The normal speakers were selected to match an average group of aphasics for age, gender and social background.

Table 10.1. Gender, age, aetiology (aetio) and months post-onset (mpo) for the aphasic subjects

Patient	Gender	Age	aetio	mpo
1	m	72	CVA	>60
2	m	45	CVA	>60
3	f	38	CVA	>60
4	m	44	CVA	12
5	m	53	CVA	12
6	m	65	CVA	5
7	f	63	CVA	>60
8	f	44	CVA	10

CVA: cerebo-vascular accident.

Materials

The test for *action naming* consists of 60 items, controlled for instrumentality and name relation with nouns.[1] The items were also controlled for word frequency and transitivity. The frequency distribution is the same among the three groups of verbs. Half of the items in each group are transitive, the other half being intransitive, each half again controlled for frequency. Because all items concern action verbs, the argument structure is either *Verb + agent, theme* (for the transitives) or *Verb + agent* (for the intransitives).

All pictures have been named correctly by at least 80% of a control group, consisting of ten neurologically unimpaired, healthy subjects who matched an average aphasia subgroup in age, gender and social background (this was not the same control group as the one that was used for the spontaneous speech analysis).

Procedure

Each action was depicted in a simple line drawing on a separate page and presented to the patient one at a time. The patient was asked to tell in one word what the person in the picture was doing.

The test started with two examples. If patients failed to give the intended reaction to an example they were corrected. After the examples, no more verbal feedback was given. There was no time limit and self-correction was allowed.

As well as assessment with this test, a spontaneous speech sample was recorded. The patients were asked to tell how their speech problems started. The normal speakers were asked to tell about their last illness to get comparable samples, especially with respect to verb tense. If this question did not elicit sufficient spontaneous speech, patients and controls were asked to tell about their professional history and their daily activities. The samples were transcribed orthographically and the length of 300 words was established according to the method of Vermeulen, Bastiaanse and van Wageningen (1989).

Scoring

For scoring action naming, the only point taken into account was whether or not the intended target (or, in a few cases, a synonym that was frequently used by the control subjects) was given.

The spontaneous speech samples were analysed with regard to verb production. For lexical analysis, the total number of verbs (= tokens) was counted. As a bare number of verbs does not give very much insight, the diversity was calculated by a type–token ratio (ttr): the number of different verbs (the types) was divided by the number of tokens, giving a ratio between 1.00 and 0.00. A high ratio means a great diversity, a low ratio implies poor diversity and, hence, low lexical content (see e.g. Vermeulen, Bastiaanse and van Wageningen, 1989).

Three other variables were taken into account, to reflect morphosyntactic and argument structure abilities. First of all, the inflection index was calculated: for each clause containing a verb, it was established whether there was a finite verb. The total number of finite verbs was divided by the total number of clauses containing a verb. Copulas and modal verbs (contrary to English, the latter are inflected for agreement in Dutch) were also considered to be finite verbs.

The number of modals and copulas was included as a separate variable, to evaluate the relationship between inflection in general and the production of these word classes that are most frequently used in their inflected form. Secondly, the argument structures of the verbs were analysed. This was done according to the method of Edwards, Garman and Knott (1993) that only takes realized arguments into account. For each verb it was counted how many internal arguments were realized (external arguments were ignored, as even in normal speech these are sometimes omitted). Only including realized arguments makes our analysis different from the ones performed by, for example, Byng and Black (1989) Thompson, Shapiro, Li and Schendel (1995) and Thompson, Lange, Schneider and Shapiro (1997). In our experience the method of Edwards, Garman and Knott (1993) is more suitable for spontaneous speech, because it is very difficult to decide on the number of arguments required. Modal verbs (*can, must* etc.) were not included in the argument-structure analysis, but copulas were considered to be verbs with one internal argument

Results

Action naming is, as expected, impaired. The results are given in Table 10.2. The mean score for the group is just under 50% correct, although there is variation in the performance.

In the spontaneous speech analysis (see Table 10.2), two lexical variables were taken into account: the number of verbs and the diversity of verbs, the latter expressed by a type–token ratio.

The agrammatics do not differ significantly from the normal controls on the number of verbs they produce in 300 words spontaneous speech (mwu test: $z = -0.58$, $p = 0.56$). Only two agrammatics fall outside the (lower side of) the normal range. The diversity of the produced verbs is

Table 10.2. Results on the action naming test and the verb analysis of spontaneous speech: number and type–token ratio (ttr) of the lexical verbs, proportion of inflected verbs (infl.) and the number of modals and copulas

	Naming	Number	ttr*	infl.*	mod+cop
Agrammatics					
Mean	29.25	23.25	0.52	0.74	11.75
sdv	9.21	9.11	0.17	0.17	6.56
Controls					
Mean	—	26.75	0.75	0.91	12.75
sdv	—	3.99	0.09	0.07	3.96

significantly lower than normal (z = –2.32, p = 0.02), showing that, although the agrammatics produce as many verbs as normal controls, these verbs express less lexical content.

The proportion of inflected verbs is significantly lower in the agrammatic group, compared to the normal speakers (z = –2.05, p = 0.04), but the number of copulas and modals is normal (z = –0.37, p = 0.71); only one agrammatic fell outside the (upper side of the) normal range.

In Table 10.3, an overview is given for the verb-argument structures that were produced.

Table 10.3. Proportion of the number of internal arguments produced with the verbs (copulas but not modals included)

	0*	1	2	Clausal
Agrammatics				
Mean	0.42	0.55	0.00	0.03
sdv	0.20	0.19	0.01	0.05
Controls				
Mean	0.24	0.67	0.05	0.04
sdv	0.06	0.05	0.04	0.05

Proportionally, agrammatics produce significantly more verbs without an internal argument and, as a consequence, fewer constructions with one or two internal arguments than normal controls (no internal arguments: z = –2.48, p = 0.01; one internal argument z = –2.53, p = 0.01, two internal arguments: z = –3.08, p = 0.00). The number of verbs with a clausal argument does not differ significantly, but is low in both groups (z = –1.04, p = 0.29). It should be noticed that agrammatics do exploit the same pattern as the normal speakers: verbs with one internal argument are produced most, followed by verbs without an internal argument, whereas verbs with two internal arguments or a clausal argument are hardly used.

Action naming in relation to verbs in spontaneous speech

To evaluate the relationship between verb retrieval in a naming task and in spontaneous speech, the correlation coefficients between the scores on the action naming test and both the number of lexical verbs and the ttr were computed. No significant correlation was found between the number of lexical verbs in spontaneous speech and action naming (rho = 0.41, p > 0.05). This is not a surprising result, because action naming is severely impaired, whereas the number of lexical verbs in spontaneous speech is normal. More remarkable, however, is that the correlation between the scores on the action naming test and the diversity of verbs in spontaneous speech (the ttr) fails to reach significance too (rho = 0.64, $p > 0.05$). When we look at the individual scores (Table 10.4) it is clear why this is the case: patients B3, B4 and B8 reach the highest scores on the action naming test (above the mean score), whereas B3 is the only one of these three who scores above mean on the type–token ratio.

Table 10.4. Individual results of the agrammatics on the action naming test, type-token ratio (ttr) and the proportion of verb inflection (infl.)

	Naming	ttr*	infl.*
1	29	0.78	0.50
2	29	0.55	0.51
3	46	0.76	0.70
4	35	0.50	0.80
5	18	0.36	0.69
6	29	0.42	0.93
7	17	0.33	0.88
8	31	0.48	0.93
Mean	29.25	0.52	0.74

The question then arises why are the ttrs of verbs low when this cannot be explained by poor verb retrieval alone? Inspection of the individual data (see Figure 10.1 and Table 10.4) demonstrates that three agrammatics (B1, B2, B3) have an above average ttr, but are poor in verb inflection; four agrammatics (B4, B6, B7, B8) show the opposite pattern: low ttrs, but above average on verb inflection; one agrammatic is poor on both variables (B5).

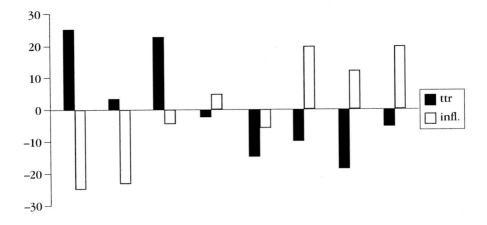

Figure 10.1. The type–token ratio (ttr) and verb inflection index (infl.) of the individual agrammatics. The x-axis is the mean score of the group, the y-axis the individual deviation × 100.

This suggests that if agrammatics show relatively normal verb inflection, a skill that is notoriously difficult for agrammatics, this is at the cost of lexical content of the verbs: the ttr drops dramatically, even if the patient is relatively good in action naming (like B4, B6 and B8). Those agrammatics who ignore verb inflections show a (close to) normal diversity of verbs in spontaneous speech. Patient B5 is poor on both variables, but his score on the action naming test is very low as well.

Patients B4, B6 and B8, whose scores are high on verb inflection, produce many modals and copulas (B8 even produces more than normal controls). These are all inflected, meaning that a large part of the inflected verbs they produce are not finite lexical verbs, but highly frequent inflected forms of modals and copulas.

This leads to the conclusion that the supposed relation between the poor performance on an action naming test and the poor production of verbs in spontaneous speech is not the one-to-one relation that has been suggested by Berndt, Mitchum, Haendiges and Sandson (1997). How can it be that Saffran, Berndt and Schwartz (1989), Bastiaanse, Jonkers and Moltmaker-Osinga (1995) and Thompson, Shapiro, Li and Schendel (1995) mention a reduced number of verbs, whereas in the present study this was not found? The reason is probably the difference in sample length for which the earlier studies did not match. Some of their patients produced fewer than 100 words, whereas others (including the normal controls) produced significantly more. Strictly speaking, it is only appropriate to compare scores on a lexical variable (like the number of verbs or a verb–noun ratio), if the samples contain an equal number of lexical units (see Vermeulen, Bastiaanse and van Wageningen, 1989). The previous studies based their claims about the reduced number of verbs on samples of unequal sample size or on samples that were matched on the number of utterances (being a grammatical rather than a lexical variable). This approach may well have obscured the results and caused the difference in results with the present study.

In summary, our first study reveals that the lexical problems concerning verbs in spontaneous speech are expressed by a low ttr, meaning that although the number of verbs produced is normal, these verbs show less variation than those of normal speakers. Those patients who are poor in verb inflection have an above average diversity of verbs. Those patients who produce an above average proportion of inflected verbs, show very little diversity in their verbs. This suggests that the low diversity of the produced verbs in this group of agrammatic aphasics is not (only) caused by poor lexical retrieval, but by a grammatical disorder that affects the ability to produce inflected verbs. If individual patients do inflect their verbs, this is always at the cost of the diversity of the verbs they produce.

Verb inflection includes at least two grammatical aspects, that is a morphological one (the grammatical morpheme) and a syntactic one (verb movement). This raises the question of whether the inflectional problems with verbs can be further fractionated.

Verb inflection: morphology vs. syntax

Syntactic background

Dutch has been analysed as an SOV language, meaning that the base-generated position of the verb is after the object, or VP-final (Koster, 1975). In the Dutch declarative matrix sentence, the finite verb has to be moved to the second position. This movement is known as *Verb Second*. In the embedded clause, however, the finite verb remains *in situ*. This is illustrated in (1) and (2), where *t* designates the canonical verb position, which is co-indexed with the Verb Second position.

1. *matrix sentence*
   de jongen leest$_i$ een boek t$_i$
   the boy reads a book

2. *embedded clause*
   (ik denk) dat de jongen een boek leest
   (I think) that the boy a book reads
   (I think that the boy reads a book)

In Figures 10.2(a) and (b) the syntactic trees picturing these clauses are given. Here it is assumed that a verb is inserted in the structure in its fully inflected form (Chomsky, 1995; for Dutch syntax, see Zwart, 1993). In the embedded clause, the finite verb remains in its base-generated position; in the matrix clause, the finite verb moves to the left. In these diagrams, the verb moves to AGRS in a simple Subject–V$_{fin}$– Object (X) matrix clause (Fig. 10.2a); the verb remains in its original position in the embedded clause, where AGRS is not lexical (Fig 10.2b).

It is the production of the inflected verb in these two positions that has been tested in this study. Several outcomes are possible, pointing to different underlying impairments. If the problems with verbs are due to an underlying morphological disorder, as, for example, suggested by Bates and Wulfeck (1989), then it is to be expected that it makes no difference in which position the inflected verb has to be produced. If, however, the disorder is syntactic in nature, verbs that have been moved are supposed to be more difficult than verbs that have not. Consequently, it is expected that verb production in the matrix clause is more difficult than in the embedded clause. Other options are open as well, for example, that production of inflected verbs in the embedded clause is more difficult than in the matrix clause, because embedding is complex in itself, or because in the Dutch embedded clause a constituent may be placed between the subject and the verb it has to agree with. Two subtests have been developed to elicit inflected verbs in the two distinct positions.

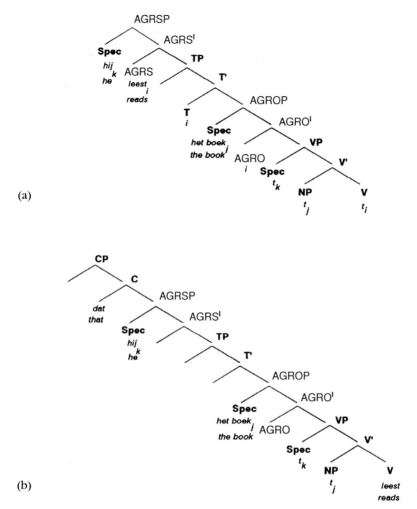

Figure 10.2. Syntactic tree of a Dutch matrix clause with Verb Second (a) and a Dutch embedded clause with the verb in final position (b).

Methods

Subjects

Eight agrammatic aphasics (5 male, 3 female) participated in this experiment; these were different patients to the ones in the first study. Again, these were 'classic' agrammatic Broca's aphasics, whose spontaneous speech was telegraphic and whose comprehension in a conversation was good. Seven patients were right-handed; they were aphasic due to a single left hemisphere stroke. One patient was left-handed; he was aphasic after a single right hemisphere stroke. The relevant data are given in Table 10.5.

Table 10.5. Gender, age, aetiology (aetio) and months post-onset (mpo) for the aphasic subjects

Patient	Gender	Age	aetio	mpo
1	m	58	CVA	6
2	m	85	CVA	3
3	m	70	CVA	13
4	f	83	CVA	>60
5	f	76	CVA	6
6	f	65	CVA	19
7	m	66	CVA	8
8	m	75	CVA	>60

CVA: cerebro-vascular accident.

Materials

The test for verb production consists of two subtests, (1) production of finite verbs in second position in matrix clauses, and (2) production of finite verbs in final position in embedded clauses. Within and among the subtests the verbs were matched for frequency and transitivity. Matching on transitivity was done because this factor may influence verb retrieval (Jonkers and Bastiaanse, 1996). All items were action verbs with similar thematic structures: an agent role for the intransitives and an agent and theme role for the transitives. The sentences were matched for constituent length, meaning that an adjunct was added in case of the intransitive verbs. This was done in view of subtest (1), in which the verb had to be produced in second position. If no adjunct is added, the second position is the final position as well, which would make the data uninterpretable. The sentences were printed under the picture, but the verb was left out (see Figure 10.3). The pictures had been named by 35 normal controls, who were selected to

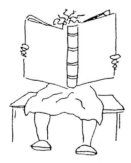
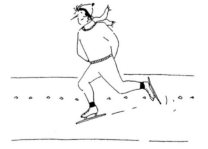

het meisje ..... een boek
the girl ..... a book

ik zie dat de jongen op de ijsbaan .....
I see that the boy on the ice rink .....
[I see that the boy ..... on the ice rink]

Figure 10.3. Two examples of the test: eliciting a finite verb in Verb Second position in the matrix clause (a) and a finite verb in final position of the embedded clause (b).

match an average aphasia group for age and social background. Each item elicited the intended responses in at least 94% of the normal controls.

Procedure

The pictures were presented one at a time. The sentence was read to the patient and at the dots, the examiner hummed three syllables. The patient was asked to complete the sentence. Of course, the patients were allowed to read the sentence themselves, but no patient was able to do so.

Each subtest started with two examples. On these items feedback was given. If patients gave a correct answer, they were encouraged. Errors were corrected until the examiner supposed that the patient understood the aim of the test. After these two examples, no more verbal feedback was given. All reactions were audio-taped and transcribed orthographically.

Scoring

First it was established whether the correct lexical item was retrieved. For these correctly retrieved items it was established whether they were correctly inflected. Only correctly retrieved items were taken into account, because we were only interested in inflection, not in lexical or phonemic errors. The proportional scores (number of correctly inflected verbs divided by the number of correctly retrieved verbs) were compared.

Results

In Table 10.6 the results are given. One patient (no. 8) did not retrieve any verbs in second position correctly and hence no proportional scores could be computed. These scores were excluded from the analysis, but they are shown here, because they reflect the general pattern.

Table 10.6. Numbers of correctly retrieved (lex+), correctly retrieved and correctly inflected (infl+) verbs and the proportion of correctly inflected verbs on the number of correctly retrieved verbs in the matrix and embedded clause

| Patient | Matrix clause (verb second) | | | Embedded clause (verb final) | | |
	lex+	infl+	prop	lex+	infl+	prop
1	6	0	0.00	10	8	0.80
2	2	0	0.00	8	4	0.50
3	5	5	1.00	9	9	1.00
4	2	0	0.00	5	4	0.80
5	8	6	0.75	10	10	1.00
6	6	2	0.33	6	5	0.83
7	5	4	0.80	6	6	1.00
8	0	0	—	4	4	1.00
Mean	4.25	2.13	0.41	8.00	6.25	0.83
sdv	2.66	2.63	0.43	2.07	2.43	0.22

Comparison of the two conditions shows that production of finite verbs in second position (in the matrix clause) is significantly more difficult than production of the same forms in clause final position (in the embedded clause) (Wilcoxon signed rank: $z = -2.12$, $p = 0.034$). All in all 22 inflectional errors were made with the correctly retrieved lexical forms. These are 13 substitutions by infinitives, eight substitutions by stems[2] and one tense error.

There is no effect for transitivity when both lexical retrieval and inflection are taken into account. Although transitive verbs seem to be somewhat easier to retrieve than intransitive verbs, the difference does not reach significance.

In summary, the data show that agrammatics encounter severe problems in producing finite verbs in Verb Second position. When the same finite forms have to be produced in the base-generated clause final position, they perform almost faultlessly, even though a construction with an embedded clause is supposed to be syntactically more complex than one without.

Several possible outcomes were mentioned above. One was that the finite verb in the embedded clause would be more difficult, because embedding as such is more complex than a simple matrix clause. Another reason why verbs in embedded clauses might have been more difficult, is that the distance between the verb and the subject it has to agree with is longer in the embedded than in the matrix clause. Clearly, these points do not play a major role, the opposite result is found, finite verbs in the embedded clause are easier to produce than those in the matrix clause. A morphological account predicts that inflected verbs are equally problematic in the matrix and the embedded clause, because finite verbs as such are difficult. The results show, however, that the production of finite verbs as such is unimpaired in agrammatic patients: they are perfectly able to use inflected verbs in the embedded clause condition. These findings exclude a morphological basis of their problems with verb inflection. A syntactic account can fully explain the data. It looks as though it is the structural position of the verb that plays a decisive role: a verb that has been moved from its base-generated position to second position is difficult to produce for these agrammatic patients.

When the results of these two studies are taken together, the conclusion is that the problems with verb production in spontaneous speech are syntactic in nature. This syntactic disorder prevents the production of finite verbs in matrix clauses (and the production of embedded clauses, see Friedmann, this book). If an agrammatic patient focuses on the production of finite verbs despite this impairment, this is directly at the cost of the diversity of the verbs produced. A patient can refrain from verb inflection and focus on lexical retrieval: in that case the lexical diversity is much better, though not always normal, given a more general lexical retrieval deficit. This choice is, of course, not a conscious one. It is even possible that individual patients shift between these options, focusing more on inflection at one time and more on lexical content at another time (see Bastiaanse, 1995).

The idea that the problems with verb production are related to verb movement, makes one wonder whether aspects associated with verb movement are impaired as well. An interesting case in this respect is negation, because negation interferes with verb movement in some languages (like English) but not in others (like Dutch). The last experiment is a cross-linguistic, explorative one on the construction of negative sentences by English and Dutch agrammatics.

Negation: head vs. specifier

Syntactic background

In order to negate a statement, two possibilities are open: sentence negation and constituent negation. Languages differ with respect to the syntactic realization of sentence negation. In English and Dutch, the negative sentence contains one NegP, with a head and a specifier. According to Ouhalla (1990) in English, NegP is situated between TP and AGRO, whereas in Dutch it is between AGRO and VP. This is a reasonable assumption, because in English, *not* precedes the verb and the object (the boy does *not* eat the apple), whereas Dutch *niet* is post-object (de jongen eet de appel *niet*, lit. the boy eats the apple *not*).

It is not only the position of NegP in the structure that is different in these two languages, the internal structure differs as well (see Figure 10.4). In English, *not* blocks movement from the verb to T and AGRS, as a consequence of the so-called *Head Movement Constraint (HMC):* head-over-head movement is not allowed and as *not* blocks movement from V to T and AGRS (cf. *the dog bites not the man), *not* is supposed to be the head of the NegP. Because the verb cannot move to T, *do*-support is needed to form a grammatical sentence (cf. the dog does not bite the man). *Does*, like other auxiliaries and modals in English, is supposed to be base-generated in T and is thus not supposed to have crossed over the head of NegP.[3]

In Dutch, the verb moves over NegP to the second position and therefore, *niet* cannot be the head of the NegP, because if it is, it has blocked movement to T. Saving the HCM, the head of NegP is supposed to be filled with an abstract morpheme (Ouhalla, 1990). Quite interesting in this respect is that in medieval Dutch, there was double negation – as in contemporary French – from which the first element, that is not used any more, clitizised with the verb. According to Ouhalla, Dutch *niet* is in the specifier as it does not interfere with verb movement.

The second type of negation is *constituent negation* (or *narrow focus negation*). In English, for example, when confronted with a picture in

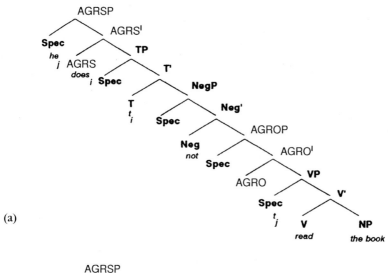

(a)

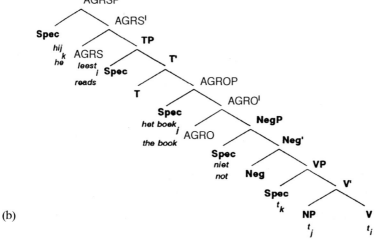

(b)

Figure 10.4. The syntactic tree of an English (a) and a Dutch (b) negative sentence (sentence negation).

which a boy is eating a banana, with an apple in his neighbourhood, one may say 'the boy eats *not* the apple, but the banana'. In sentences like this, 'not' is supposed to be generated VP-internal, as shown in Figure 10.5. In order to interpret or produce this negation, the constituent has to be moved to or via NegP, if not in overt syntax, then at LF (see Haegeman, 1995). As the verb is allowed to move to T and AGRS over this negated constituent in English and Dutch, the specifier of NegP is supposed to be the landing site in both languages; otherwise, the filled functional head of the NegP would block verb movement to T and AGRS. Both in English and in Dutch, constituent negation is marked and only used to express oppositions.

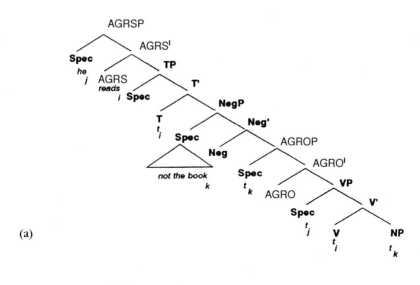

(a)

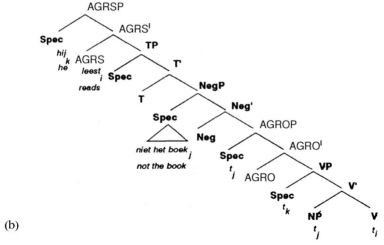

(b)

Figure 10.5. The syntactic tree of an English (a) and a Dutch (b) sentence with constituent negation. In English, movement of the verb and the object to T, AGRS and AGRO respectively is covert; it is therefore reasonable to assume that movement of the negated object to NegP is also at LF.

It is the interference with verb movement that makes negation an interesting subject to investigate in agrammatism. As was concluded from the two other studies, verb movement is complicated for agrammatics and therefore it is hypothesized that negation in English, where it is related to verb movement, will be more difficult than negation in Dutch. In order to test this hypothesis, a sentence anagram test was developed and five patients were tested on their abilities to construct negative sentences as compared to affirmative ones.

Methods

Subjects

Five agrammatic Broca's aphasics participated in this explorative study. The relevant data are given in Table 10.7. Two were native speakers of English (one Canadian and one British English) and three were native speakers of Dutch. Five age, sex and education matched normal speakers were included as control subjects, two were British, three were Dutch.

Table 10.7. Gender, age, aetiology (aetio) and months post-onset (mpo) for the aphasic subjects (English and Dutch)

Patient	Gender	Age	aetio	mpo
English				
1	f	65	CVA	>60
2	f	67	CVA	>60
Dutch				
1	m	68	CVA	16
2	m	46	CVA	18
3	f	35	CVA	16

CVA: cerebro-vascular accident.

Materials

A sentence anagram test was developed, consisting of 30 items. Three sentence types were tested: actives, passives and sentences in the present perfect tense (10 items each). Half of the items were negative sentences, the other half were affirmative controls. Only sentences that could be literally translated were included, in order to keep the results in the two languages comparable. The constituents were printed on individual cards; the *by*-phrase in the passive sentence was printed with the belonging NP on a single card, in order not to complicate the task by letting the patient choose which NP is the agent or the theme. An example of a sentence anagram is:

> [the mouse] [is] [not] [caught] [by the cat]
> [de muis] [wordt] [niet] [door de kat] [gevangen]
> (the mouse is not caught by the cat)

Notice that the difference between the two languages interferes with the task: the English active sentences have one card more than the Dutch, as in English *does* is needed. It was chosen not to give an extra card (e.g. an adverb) to the Dutch in this condition to equal the number of cards, as this would have changed the design of the experiment. This difference only held for the active sentences, not for the passives and for the sentences in perfect present tense.

Procedure and scoring

The cards were presented to the patients in pseudo-randomized order and they were asked to form a sentence using all cards. Two examples were given and patients were corrected if the sentence was not the one intended. After the two examples, no more verbal feedback was given. Self-corrections were allowed. The final reaction was written down and analysed with respect to syntactic correctness and the position of the negation. In the active sentences (both perfect and imperfect tense) errors in which the order of the NPs was reversed were ignored.

Results

Both the English- and the Dutch-speaking control subjects put the sentences in the correct order without any hesitance. Counting the errors of the Dutch agrammatics raised some problems as many of the negative sentences were formed with constituent negation, which is perfectly grammatical, though marked, in Dutch. None of the Dutch control subjects used this construction. In order to score as conservatively as possible, constituent negation was counted as an error. The results of the individual agrammatics are given in Table 10.8.

Table 10.8. Proportion of correctly constructed negative and affirmative sentences

Patient	Negative sentences			Affirmative sentences		
	Active	Passive	Perfect	Active	Passive	Perfect
English						
1	0.00	0.00	0.00	1.00	0.80	1.00
2	0.20	0.00	0.20	1.00	0.80	1.00
Dutch						
1	1.00	0.00	1.00	1.00	1.00	1.00
2	0.20	0.60	0.20	1.00	0.60	0.60
3	0.20	1.00	0.00	1.00	1.00	1.00

The English patients are significantly better in constructing affirmative sentences than negative sentences (Wilcoxon test: $z = -2.12, p = 0.034$), for Dutch the difference is very close to significant (Wilcoxon test: $z = -1.94, p = 0.053$). Further quantitative analysis shows that the English patients are significantly more impaired in constructing negative sentences than the Dutch (mwu test: $z = -1.99, p = 0.046$). The difference between the two languages on the affirmative sentences is not significant (mwu test: $z = -0.15, p = 0.879$).

Qualitative analysis shows that the behaviour of the five patients in constructing negative sentences is strikingly similar. The majority of the errors concern constituent negation (English: no.1 87%, no.2 100%; Dutch: no.1 100%, no.2 60%, no.3 78%). In English this leads to ungrammatical sentences like 'the boy does congratulate not the girl' and marked sentences like 'the dinner is cooked not by the man'. Interestingly, the English agrammatics use *does* correctly in the active sentences, although they negate the object. In Dutch, the sentences with constituent negation are all grammatical, but marked and not produced by the control subjects (and therefore counted as errors).

In summary, there are two major findings: first, the English patients are more impaired than the Dutch on the negative sentences; secondly, all patients tend to use constituent negation when they make errors, even if this results in ungrammatical sentences, as in English.

It is not very plausible that the quantitative difference is caused by the fact the Dutch are overall less impaired than the English: the English and the Dutch perform equally well on the affirmative control sentences. A ceiling effect obscuring a quantitative difference is not very likely either: three out of the five patients make at least one error and the worst performing patient is Dutch. Therefore, we would like to suggest that it is the status of NegP that influences the patients' performance. When the negation is in the specifier position, as Dutch *niet*, it seems to generate fewer problems than when it has the status of functional head, as English *not*. The question then arises why this may be the case. Negation as a functional head may be more difficult, because it interferes with verb movement. That is, the fact that negation as a functional head blocks verb movement to T and AGRS in English may make the production of negative sentences more complicated and may result in the construction of ungrammatical sentences. Construction of negative sentences by Dutch agrammatics is not perfect, even though the negation word is in the specifier of NegP, but it is significantly better than in English agrammatics and it results in marked, rather than ungrammatical sentences. Nevertheless, qualitatively there is no difference between the patient groups: if they make errors, it is by using constituent negation. Why would agrammatics apply constituent negation instead of sentential negation? For English it is clear: although the negated constituent has to be moved to NegP, its landing site is in the specifier, and not in Neg. Therefore, constituent negation does not interfere with verb movement: the verb can move via NegP to T and AGRS: *the boy eats* <u>*not*</u> *the banana (but the apple)* . It is unclear, however, why the Dutch agrammatics resort to constituent negation, because there is no interference with verb movement in the first place. Apparently, there is more to sentence negation than interference with verb movement that makes it difficult to handle for agrammatics.

Although one should keep in mind that both the number of patients and the number of items in this experiment are low, the difference between English and Dutch agrammatics seems to indicate that performance on the negative sentence varies with respect to the syntactic status of the negation.

General discussion

The three studies show that agrammatic production is seriously compromised with respect to verb movement and related issues (inflection and negation). In spontaneous speech, verb inflection is reduced, but if an individual patient uses many (though not a normal amount of) inflected verbs, this reduces the diversity of the verbs produced. The problems with verb inflection seem to be syntactic, rather than morphological in nature: in an experimental task, agrammatics are impaired in their production of verbs that have been moved from their canonical position, whereas production of finite verbs in base-generated position is almost perfect. The last study demonstrates that functional heads that are related to verb movement (like negation in English) are also difficult to handle.

This central role of verb movement in agrammatic production is remarkable, because it has been suggested that verb movement does not play a significant role in grammatical judgment, that is, that agrammatic Broca's aphasics correctly judge the (un)grammaticality of sentences in which verb movement was applied (Grodzinsky and Ballogh, 1998). And for production, Bastiaanse and Van Zonneveld (1998) showed in a previous explorative study that Dutch agrammatics are sensitive to the relation between verb inflection and verb position: in spontaneous speech, the clausal word order is either *finite verb - object* or *object - nonfinite verb*. Ungrammatical word order, like *hij lezen boek* (Verb Second with a non-finite verb) or *hij boek leest* (matrix clause–final finite verb) was not observed. Taking the results of these studies together, it must be concluded that although verb movement yields difficulties for agrammatic aphasics, they are very well aware of the fact that in matrix clauses finite verbs should be in Verb Second position and non-finite verbs in clause final position, even though these verbs in Verb Second position are very hard for them to produce.

The negation experiment revealed that functional heads related to verb movement give rise to problems as well. The production of *not* as a functional head is evaded by applying constituent negation, but this cannot be explained by the relation to verb movement alone. Dutch agrammatics use the same strategy, although to a significantly smaller extent, although the Dutch negation *niet* is supposed to be in the specifier of NegP.

This leads to two questions. The first is whether the difference between the influence of the status of negation as a specifier or as a head can be found in other languages. We are currently testing Afrikaans, Spanish, Norwegian and Hungarian speaking agrammatics to find an answer to this question. The second question is whether other word-classes that are related to verb movement are affected as well. To answer this, we evaluated the production of determiners and pronouns in relation to verb production. This (explorative) study also suggests that impaired production of these word classes is closely related to the presence of their case assigners, that is, the Verb (that assigns dative and accusative Case to the indirect and direct object) and its inflection (that assigns nominative Case to the subject) (Ruigendijk, Bastiaanse and Van Zonneveld, 1998).

We would therefore like to conclude that the role of the verb in agrammatic production seems to be crucial: many of the classic characteristics of telegraphic speech may be closely connected to the production of verbs in general and of moved verbs in particular: little variety in verb production (or relying on light verbs, as mentioned by Berndt, Mitchum, Haendiges and Sandson, 1997), lack of verb inflection, marked or ungrammatical structures (like constituent negation in English), omission of determiners and pronouns and maybe others. This is all in line with the prediction of Grodzinsky (1990), who mentioned that functional heads are omitted from surface structure in agrammatic speech. Nevertheless, we would like to narrow this to a hypothesis that predicts that mainly those functional heads that are related to verb movement are vulnerable in agrammatic production, whereas others, like *does* in English active, negative sentences and modals and copulas in Dutch matrix clauses are retained.

Notes

[1] Instrumental verbs are defined as the names of those actions for which a man-made instrument is required (e.g. *to saw*, *to cut*). In Dutch, as in other languages, instrumental verbs may or may not be related in name to the instrument. In the test, 20 items are non-instrumental verbs (e.g. *to climb*), 20 items are instrumental verbs without name relation (e.g. *to stir*) and 20 items are instrumental with a name relation (e.g. *to ski*).

[2] Notice that in Dutch the stem is different from the infinitival form. The infinitival form is stem + /en/. The stem is the same form as the first-person singular, present tense, whereas the non-finite form is the same as the plural, present tense. For this reason only the third-person singular was used (stem + t in Dutch) in conditions in which the verb had to be inflected.

[3] For Dutch it is assumed that auxiliaries and modals are generated within the VP; in matrix clauses they are moved to the second position, like lexical verbs. In embedded clauses, the auxiliaries and modals remain clause final (e.g. ik zie dat hij het boek gelezen heeft, lit. I see that he the book read has).

Chapter 11
A clinical assessment of verbs in an agrammatic patient

SUSAN EDWARDS

Introduction

Traditional, clinical descriptions of Broca's aphasia comment on the non-fluent effortful speech, the short utterances, frequent pauses and word-finding difficulties where content words are relatively well preserved compared with function words. The typically short utterances are said to be constructed around major lexical-class words (Garman, 1990). Such descriptions act as a 'rough and ready', useful clinical characterization but offer nothing in terms of furthering our knowledge of lexical and syntactic deficits found in this disorder or in relating the phenomena observed to current linguistic theories. Comparatively recent psycholinguistic research has made some progress in establishing more detailed characterizations of agrammatism and in formulating descriptions within recognized linguistic frameworks. For example, Friedmann and Grodzinsky (1997) have produced a characterization of agrammatism within the context of the Minimalist programme. The authors consider data from a Hebrew speaking aphasic in which tense but not agreement is impaired

Traditional descriptions of aphasia have also been challenged in terms of the details observed. Despite the relative preservation of 'major lexical classes' noted in such descriptions, for example, it is increasingly recognized that within the relatively well-preserved lexical classes, verbs may be more vulnerable than nouns in Broca's aphasia (Saffran, Schwartz and Marin, 1980; Miceli, Mazzuchi, Menn and Goodglass, 1983). Some findings are contradictory and it must therefore be assumed that verb deficits are not an essential feature of the Broca's aphasia and variations may be found across patients (Berndt, Mitchum, Haendiges and Sandson, 1997a) and languages (Chen and Bates, 1998).

As a result of such publications, clinicians are increasingly aware that an agrammatic patient may have problems with lexical verb retrieval as well as the more well-attested syntactic deficits associated with verb morphology. Unfortunately, published tests offer little guidance as to how a clinician might test a patient's ability to retrieve verbs. Although there are clinical tests available to test noun production, material for testing verb production is extremely sparse. This chapter contains a report on a clinical investigation of a verb deficit in one aphasic speaker using a range of published and unpublished procedures. There were two purposes for the assessments. First the aim was to see if a verb deficit was present and if so whether the number of arguments associated with the verb affected verb retrieval; secondly, we wished to compare verb retrieval using the traditional format of clinical tests with verb retrieval in spontaneous, connected speech.

Verbs in agrammatic speech

Chen and Bates (1998) summarize a number of possible explanations as to why verbs might be more 'difficult' than nouns for some aphasic patients. Their explanations include the assumption that at some level of mental representation, verbs carry semantic information as well as syntactic information (inflectional morphology and subcategorization) so that, presumably, verb impairment may arise as a result of impairment at either or both levels of representation. Verbs are 'critical to sentence structure as they help specify the relations between words in a sentence' (Shapiro and Levine, 1990: 22). The semantic and syntactic information carried imposes certain restrictions and ensures that the intact system will only produce well-formed (semantically and syntactically) sentences. The syntactic constraints of subcategorization specify the types of syntactic environment a verb requires whereas the argument structure of a verb specifies the number of participants a verb must or may be associated with (Shapiro, 1997: 261). Work by Shapiro, Zurif and Grimshaw (1987) suggested that, for normal language users, the complexity of a verb can be defined by the number of different argument structures with which it is associated. (In these cross-modal lexical decision tasks, reaction time was taken to indicate degree of verb complexity.) Shapiro and Levine (1990: 45), following up this work, found that agrammatic aphasics performed in a similar way to their normal controls. The *pattern* of reaction time, longer reaction time for more complex verbs, was the same for the agrammatic subjects and control subjects. They therefore concluded that the agrammatic subjects, like the normal controls, were sensitive to all possible argument structures of the verbs tested whereas fluent aphasic speakers, who had a different pattern of reaction times, 'were not sensitive to the argument structure information represented with verbs'. The authors concluded that 'access to the lexicon and to a verb's thematic information is normal for agrammatic Broca's patients: it is the post-activation stage, the assignment of thematic role which contributes to comprehension problems in these patients (p. 40).

Given these results and the authors' conclusions, we might expect agrammatic patients to show good understanding of verbs and the argument structures required. Furthermore, this 'awareness' (which of course is not taken to be a conscious awareness), might impact on verb production in that verbs which are more complex (in terms of number of associated argument structure), are more difficult for agrammatic speakers to produce.

However, some caution is needed in interpreting and extrapolating from these results. Shapiro and Levine note that the protocols they employed used simple canonical sentences and the findings might not hold for more complex sentence structures. Secondly, inspection of their results show that their Broca's aphasic subjects, although showing a parallel pattern to the normal controls, were slower in reaction times especially in the tasks involving verbs with complex argument structure arrangements. This could be interpreted as evidence that verb processing demanded greater cognitive resources within the impaired system, put simply, the task was more difficult for the aphasic subjects and was executed at the cost of time. Thirdly, we cannot assume that the results obtained on a processing task in experimental conditions can be matched by tasks examining output (or, indeed, naturalistic connected speech). The task did not require subjects to say verbs as single words or within sentences so there is no way of knowing whether these aphasic subjects could produce the verbs that they were processing, albeit slowly. Access to the verb's argument structures need not, presumably, guarantee ability to say the word. Finally, the difficulty exposed in the experiment may be with the task as much as the complexity of the sentences to be parsed: a longer reaction time in the cross-modal decision in the experimental task, has been shown elsewhere. Zurif, Swinney, Prather, Solomon and Bushell (1993: 452) considering Broca's patients' sensitivity to prime-target relations note that 'their priming seems to be temporally protracted' and that lexical activation in priming tasks 'seems to have a slower-than-normal time course'. So a Broca's patient 'normal access to the lexicon' may supply the full representation of the verb's argument structures, although the rate of access is slow compared with non-brain damaged subjects. 'Lexical access' may not, then, be taken to predict normal verb production.

These consideration may help to reconcile the above claims of full access to verbs and their argument structures with the well-attested findings that at least some agrammatic speakers have problems accessing verbs in single-word tests as well as sentence construction (Bastiaanse, 1991; Breedin and Martin, 1996; Berndt, Mitchum, Haendiges and Sanderson, 1997a,b.; Jonkers, 1998). Agrammatic speakers with verb deficits either do not have 'full activation' for all verbs, or have 'full activation' at a level of mental representation prior to activation of the phonological form of the verb. If the first is true, then one would expect performance to vary across verbs: this was not reported by Shapiro and

Levine. The second explanation would lead us to expect better clinical performance on tasks requiring processing/selection/comprehension of verbs than those requiring production of verbs. Even fairly limited clinical tests could highlight a comprehension/production difference in ability.

Further predictions might be made. If the prolonged reaction times of the agrammatic subjects in Shapiro and Levine experiments signify some problem of resource allocation at the moment of verb processing, then we might expect delayed responses in clinical tasks involving verb activation. Given that varying structural properties of verbs (in terms of the number of associated argument structures) make different demands in experimental conditions, then we can predict that this effect will be seen in clinical tests: we can predict that the complexity of a verb will be a factor in verb activation for both comprehension and production tasks.

Unfortunately, it has been found that 'sensitivity to argument structure' is not manifested in a straightforward way. Tasks which compare an aphasic's ability to access verbs with differing argument structures do not necessarily expose the predicted bias (i.e. verbs with more, rather than fewer arguments will be harder to activate). Most importantly, for the clinician, we cannot assume that the predicted bias will be manifested by all patients or in all tasks. Recent research suggests that what might appear to be less complex verbs, i.e. those associated with one argument, are not necessarily easier for aphasic speakers to produce in all tasks. Jonkers and Bastiaanse (1996) found that for their group of ten Broca's aphasic speakers, transitive verbs were easier to name than intransitive verbs, Jonkers (1998 and this volume) found that his group of 15 Broca's patients were better at naming transitive verbs than intransitive although there was variation within the group on a sentence production tasks and Gottfried, Menn and Holland (1997) found that a group of aphasic speakers were better at repeating transitive verbs than intransitive verbs (verbs were matched for frequency in all tasks). Clinicians might, then, need to investigate whether verb retrieval is associated with the number of argument structures required, bearing in mind that Shapiro and Levine found processing time increased as the number of different *structural arrangements* associated with a verb increased rather than just the *number* of argument structures.

There are some data to support the notion that some aphasic speakers will show, relative to normal speakers, a preference for verbs that take fewer than three arguments. Byng (1988) claimed that her agrammatic patient used fewer complex verbs (where number of arguments was the metric). Thompson, Shapiro, Li, and Schendel (1995), although finding that Broca's aphasic patients and normal controls produced a similar hierarchy of verb types in narrative and conversational discourse, did find some differences in verb use. The aphasic speakers were less successful using 'complex' verbs producing significantly more obligatory one-place verbs and optional two-place verbs. The normal subjects produced significantly more obligatory three-place, complement and phrasal verbs. There was no difference in the number of two-place verbs produced. Additionally, compared with the controls, there was a reduction of correctly produced different verbs. This finding is in line with the experimental findings reported above if we can conceive that in some way, Broca's patients can limit the use of verbs to those with fewer arguments. Restriction of verbs according to argument structure would impact on the range of the diversity of lexical verbs used although these two aspects may dissociate (Edwards and Bastiaanse, 1997).

Berndt, Mitchum, Haendiges and Sanderson (1997b) found a number of dissociations between different types of verb deficits in a group of 11 aphasics. For example, whereas the ability to produce verbs was not related to proficiency in the use of bound and free grammatical morphemes, it was strongly correlated with several measures of sentence structure elaboration. Five of their subjects were said to be especially dependent on 'light' verbs. For these patients, the frequent use of such verbs indicated to the authors that the patients had retained their sensitivity to the need for a verb and the ability to constrict a sentence around some type of verb (p. 130) but the range of lexical types available was reduced. So difficulty with verb retrieval does not necessarily result in problems with sentence production as it would seem that an aphasic speaker may be able to deploy a reduced range of verbs yet achieve a normal proportion of, at least, main clauses. However, there is a strong likelihood that reduced access to verbs will affect sentence production as well as the ability to convey meaning.

Clinical implications of published findings such as those briefly reviewed above, are not transparent, nor does the research indicate how best to proceed with assessment or therapy. For a clinician, faced with an agrammatic patient whom they suspect has problems with verb retrieval, there are two important initial questions. What is the nature of the deficit and which assessment procedures will be the most efficient to use in terms of information gained vs. time invested? The somewhat conflicting research findings suggest that clinicians need to use a range of procedures, as results (and therefore conclusion about the extent and nature of the verb deficit) have been shown to vary depending on procedure used. For example, certain subgroups of agrammatic aphasic speakers are better at verb production in sentences rather than single word tasks, although for others, the reverse is true (Jonkers, this volume).

The clinical assessment reported in this chapter focuses on two features associated with verb retrieval, the lexical diversity of verbs used (that is, straighforwardly, the number of different lexical verbs produced in a test or used in spontaneous speech) and the influence of argument structure on verb retrieval. Deficits associated with these features have important clinical implications. For example, if the range of lexical verbs used is reduced, is it sufficient to focus therapy on verb retrieval regardless of associated argument structures? Or is it expedient to encourage the use of less complex verbs (in terms of number of arguments associated with the verb) before the more complex? Is it harder, for example, to construct sentences using verbs that take two, three or sentential arguments than to construct sentences with intransitive verbs? Given that the most common type of verb used by normal speakers and aphasics (Thompson, Shapiro, Li and Schendel, 1995; Bastiaanse, Edwards and Kiss, 1996) are two-place verbs, should therapy focus on the use of these, even though they might appear more complex than intransitive verbs? Indeed, there are claims that therapy can gainfully be focused on heightening the aphasic speaker's awareness of argument structure and procedures to examine the role of verb argument structures have been proposed (Byng and Black, 1989). More recently, it has been proposed that therapists working on noun production might gainfully examine the affect of argument structure (Whitworth, 1995a) so a clinician might look for the effect of noun production when considering therapy focused on verb production.

Before any decisions about therapy can be made, it is necessary to assess the patient. The first step is to decide on which assessment procedures to use. In this study it was possible to use some new tests which are being developed for use with English-speaking patients to supplement more familiar clinical tests. Additionally, samples of spontaneous connected speech were collected for analyses. If verb production varies depending on whether the target in a test is a single-word or sentence, then it would seem important to examine the effect of connected text on verb retrieval. The testing, although motivated by the relevant literature, was conducted within the usual clinical restraints. We will see how far the results confirm performance predicted by the experimental work and consider whether the data collected within clinical conditions can give information about the nature of the deficit.

The subject and past history

Past history

The subject of this study is LE a young 29-year-old, unmarried woman, who had been a nurse on a neurosurgical ward. Eight months before the testing reported in this chapter she had sustained a left frontal cerebral infarct. A CT scan showed swelling in the left hemisphere with low-density area in the frontal region. An MRI scan showed evidence of acute middle cerebral artery territory infarction or ischemis. Further investigations failed to show a cause of the infarct. Immediately after the incident, the patient had swallowing difficulties and feeding was via a naso-gastric tube for 12 days. Voice production was impaired and there was evidence of comprehension deficits in both spoken and written language. Following the removal of the naso-gastric tube there was slow improvement in speech and more rapid improvement in comprehension.

Four weeks post-onset her comprehension had improved so that she was able to score 28/38 on a single-word synonym judgment task, 38/48 on a lexical decision task involving derivational and inflectional morphology, and 19/23 on a sentence-comprehension task involving both directional and non-directional verbs. She had speech and language therapy several times a week first during her time as an in-patient in a district hospital and then as an out-patient at a rehabilitation unit. Although speech and language therapy notes had been kept, a record of detailed testing was not available.

Current status at time of testing

At 8 months post-onset, the time of this report, LE presented as a Broca's aphasic and was described by her therapists as agrammatic. She had slow speech which comprised single words or short utterances with pauses for word searching or the correct grammatical verb form. Comprehension appeared to be good although she did occasionally ask for repetition so whether she could be regarded as a 'true' agrammatic patient depends on whether asyntactic comprehension is considered to be an essential diagnostic feature. Most agrammatic aphasic patients have a comprehension problem with certain sentence structures but it is not always the case (Kolk, Van Grunsven and Keyser, 1985): this is sometimes acknowledged (Zurif, Swinney, Prather, Solomon and Bushell, 1993) and has recently been exemplified (Friedmann and Grodzinsky, 1997). Such cases may be unusual or outliers (Zurif, Swinney, Prather, Solomon and Bushell, 1993) or may constitute a subtype. Grodzinsky (1991) has argued robustly for the entity of agrammatism stating clearly and logically that the severity or frequency of a feature is not paramount. The issue of symptom reduction over time is important to keep in mind when reviewing the test data discussed below.

Planning the assessment

The assessments were to provide an up-to-date account of one aspect of LE's language abilities, her ability to produce verbs. In trying to assess aphasic language, it is important for a clinician to consider how far traditional clinical tests of single-word and sentence production are a true reflection of speech production. Clinicians may elect to sample spontaneous speech (there are several published procedures for analysing speech samples), but all take considerably more time than single-word or sentence-based tests. So if the latter are good indicators of language ability, then, despite their apparent lack of ecological validity, they can be seen as a relatively quick way of collecting information to inform therapy and as a way of checking progress. If, however, performance varies with different procedures, then inferences must be more circumspect.

It was clear that LE had problems constructing sentences and that verbs were difficult to retrieve although the extent of the problem was not known. Research suggests that there are various factors which might influence retrieval, including argument structure so this was one aspect to explore. Additionally, the relationship between performance on clinical tests compared with spontaneous speech was of interest. It was decided, therefore, to explore the severity of the observed verb retrieval deficit compared with noun retrieval and to consider whether the number of arguments associated with a verb, influenced verb retrieval. Testing would include the analysis of speech samples as well as clinical tests.

Samples of connected speech data were collected and analysed to produce a profile of grammatical structures used and types and tokens of lexical verbs were logged to give an index of verb diversity. The verb counts would allow a crude comparison to be made between success in producing verbs in response to picture stimuli and verbs produced in connected speech. Picture material was used for the single-word and sentence tests, in line with current clinical practice. In the work reported by Berndt, Mitchum, Haendiges and Sanderson (1997b: 78), none of their 11 subjects showed a significant difference in naming actions shown on video compared with naming line drawings. Their report gives some credence to this more practical mode of testing. Descriptions and results of the investigations will be given for each type of test.

Testing comprehension

Tests of verb comprehension

Although the focus of the investigation was to be on LE's output, it was important to check whether there was a residual difficulty in comprehension. Should errors occur, it would be possible to search for argument structure influence. Furthermore, it has been suggested (for example, by Berndt, Mitchum, Haendiges and Sanderson, 1997a) that a deficit of both comprehension and production of verbs would indicate a deficit at the conceptual level. Intact comprehension but impaired production would indicate a difficulty with accessing. This might involve an inability to access the verb with the correct meaning or correct phonological form or the associated argument structures. If, however, comprehension seems to be intact and the claims of Shapiro and colleagues are correct, good comprehension of verbs ought to be associated with access to correct argument structure. Furthermore, if verbs are accessed with associated argument structures then sentence structure should not be compromised.

Three short tests were given. Two were from The Verb Expression and Comprehension Test for Aphasia: VECTA (Jonkers and Bastiaanse, 1994). The two sections used tested comprehension of verbs given as single words and comprehension of verbs within a sentence. The tests were originally devised and normed for use with Dutch speakers. The version reported on in this paper is an experimental English version. The third test was taken from The Psycholinguistic Assessment of Language in Aphasia: PALPA (Kay, Lesser and Coltheart, 1992) and tested comprehension of sentences with a range of syntactic structures. An agrammatic patient would be expected to fail on some sentences.

Results of verb comprehension tests

LE showed no difficulty with accessing meanings of verbs given as single words. She showed slightly more difficulty with sentence comprehension although her score was probably within normal limits (no norms are given by the authors for this subtest). Results are displayed in Table 11.1: non-aphasic subjects would be expected to score at or close to 100%. There was no difference in the score on the sentence comprehension test which comprised simple active sentences (VECTA) and the test which consisted of sentences with a range of syntactic structures (PALPA).

Table 11.1. Results of comprehension tests

1. Selecting verbs*	60/60 (100%)
2. Sentence-picture matching:*	58/60 (97%)
3. Sentence comprehension:**	58/60 (97%)

* VECTA (Jonkers and Bastiaanse, 1994).
** PALPA 55 (Kay, Lesser and Coltheart, 1992).

The subject, LE responded rapidly and accurately to the single-word test. She also had an impressive score on the sentence comprehension tests and so would, as far as these tests show, seem to have recovered comprehension.

Errors in comprehension tasks

However, although LE's scores were high on the sentence comprehension, she did make errors on both tests of sentence comprehension and she had an extended response time. She responded slowly and cautiously to items, pausing for some items and whispering to herself as she considered various options. This behaviour suggests that processing was slow (as predicted) and that she was aware of the need to monitor and self-correct. The two errors made were probably not significant in terms of her over-all score but her delayed response time and her need to rehearse and self-monitor suggested that she had some problems with sentence processing which had not fully recovered. Problems with sentence processing would be expected of an agrammatic patient. Observation of her performance suggested that she was unable to give the rapid and accurate responses one would expect of a non-aphasic subject. Her slow response time may be indicative of the processing load as discussed above although no comparison was made between the response times on the two different sentence comprehension tests.

In discussing the PALPA subtest with the patient, LE revealed that she was, at times, either unsure of the thematic role played by noun phrases or unsure of the exact meaning of certain verbs. On balance, her responses on this test and her attempted explanations suggested that her difficulty was not with thematic role assignment *per se* (as suggested by Shapiro and Levine, 1990) but more to do with activating the meaning of the verb. For example, she was unsure which picture portrayed the meaning of *pull* vs. *push* (which might be taken as evidence of problems with role assignment) but she was also unsure which picture conveyed *approach* and she indicated that she wasn't sure of the meaning of *suggesting*. Although open to other possible interpretations, her explanations, given via incomplete phrases, supplemented by plenty of gesture, pointing to various options and shaking her head with a variety of facial expressions, seemed to be related to accessing a precise *meaning* of a verb we might assume she would have known pre-morbidly. So, although she scored within normal limits, she did not respond with the same confidence and speed that might be expected given her previous education and occupation and her performance indicated some problems with accessing precise meaning for certain verbs.

Testing verb production in single-word and sentence tests

LE's most obvious difficulties were with language production. A range of clinical tests were given and several samples of spontaneous speech were recorded for analysis. Clinical tests comprised naming actions, constructing sentences and describing pictures with and without a spoken model given by the examiner.

Single-word tasks

The VECTA Action Naming Test was used in which the patient is required to name a series of black and white line drawings depicting various actions. For comparison, two object-naming tests, the VECTA Object Naming Test and the Boston Naming Test (Kaplan, Goodglass and Weintraub, 1983), both of which use black and white drawings, were given. The results are displayed in Table 11.2. The Dutch version of the Object Naming Test and the Action Naming Test were matched for frequency but it is not yet known whether these values hold for English speakers: English norms are not yet available. The Boston Naming Test has more low frequency items than the VECTA even though the overall mean frequency for the Boston and the VECTA Object Naming Test is similar. The score for the Boston Naming Test is for those items which were named immediately and accurately. A further four items were named correctly after latencies of greater than 5 seconds: most other errors were closely related either phonologically or semantically to the target.

Table 11.2. Results of single-word tests

1. Boston Naming Test: (object naming)	37/60	(0.61)
2. VECTA Object naming	36/60	(0.60)
3. VECTA Action naming	16/60	(0.27)

Results of single-word verb production compared with object naming

The scores on the single-word tests highlight the problem LE had with accessing open class words and indicate that verbs were harder to access than nouns. (Non-aphasic speakers could be expected to score at or near 100%.) There was no significant difference between the number of correct items on the two tests of object naming but a significance difference between the Action Naming Test and both of the Object Naming Tests (df = 1, p < 0.001). Frequency cannot account for this difference as the two VECTA tests had been matched for frequency and although there are differences in frequency values of the items in the two object naming tests, this did not seem to affect her score. Berndt, Mitchum, Haendiges and Sanderson (1997a: 79) found that although word frequency does have an effect for some aphasic speakers, the word class difference (noun/verb) is a stronger influencing factor. If we take the above test data then we can draw the same conclusion for LE, verbs were more difficult to activate than nouns on these single-word production tasks.

Errors in action naming

Although achieving a low score, LE demonstrated that she had some semantic knowledge available for most targets. When she failed she was often able to indicate that she had some representation of the meaning available by miming the activity depicted and/or producing an associated noun. So for the target *filing* where the picture showed a girl filing her nails, LE said *nails* and mimed the action. Similar mimed responses plus an associated noun were obtained for *throwing* (where she produced *ball*) and *chopping* (where she produced *axe*). Other attempts included miming only (target *sieving*) or the production of a semantically associated noun without the mimed action; *snow* for *skiing*; *bicycle* for *cycling*; *camera* for *photographing*.

An alternative interpretation could be that these errors do not indicate that LE had a semantic representation of the target verb but resulted from naming objects depicted in the stimulus pictures. Other errors, when incorrect but semantically related verbs were produced, are probably better examples of relatively preserved representation, for example, she produced *wash* for *wringing; row* for *sailing* and *swim* for *diving*. However, we have argued above that the confusions and hesitations shown in the tests for single-word comprehension indicated that access to precise semantic representation was not always available. Although this type of data cannot be used to determine whether or not semantic representation was preserved for the items she was unable to say, the errors made on the single-word naming tests do suggest that either semantic representation was damaged (but for very few items) or she occasionally had difficulty, perhaps because of the nature of the task, in accessing the semantic representation.

Effect of argument structure

What of the lexico-syntactic information within the verb's representation, the associated argument structure? LE's poor score on the Action Naming test (27%) was further examined to explore the possibility that the number of arguments associated with a verb might have influenced her performance. If information about the number of arguments required was retained, would verbs which require two arguments be more difficult to access than those requiring one? The list of verbs used for the verb test contained a number of words such as *dobbelen* and *badmintonnen* which although a single lexical item in Dutch, translated into English as a phrase *playing with dice* or *playing badminton*. The list was pruned and such words were omitted from this analysis. The remaining 50 items were then considered for argument structure: 20 were one-place verbs and 30 were obligatory two-place verbs. Those named correctly were 4/20 (20%) one-place verbs and 12/30 (40%) of the two-argument verbs. This suggests that the additional lexical information required by the verb (the arguments), and depicted in the stimulus picture might be beneficial in the process of verb retrieval (Jonkers and Bastiaanse, 1996).

Sentence construction tasks

In addition to having problems with accessing words, LE had difficulties with sentence construction. Her spontaneous speech was typically slow, often effortful and sentences were frequently abandoned. LE's ability to produce a verb within a sentence was tested to explore whether the additional requirement of sentence construction would impact on her ability to produce verbs. The VECTA Sentence Construction subtest was used. As can be seen (Table 11.3), this task proved to be less difficult than the single-word naming task in terms of total number of correctly produced verbs. There was also a difference in the proportion of correctly produced verbs depending on the argument structure associated with the verb. The patient, LE, had more difficulty constructing sentences using verbs taking two arguments than constructing sentences with intransitive verbs. Whereas we have speculated that the additional pictorial information for the transitive verbs may have assisted her in the single-word task, this did not seem to be the case when the task demanded a sentence to be constructed (see Jonkers, this volume). In this test, the additional demand of sentence construction had a greater detrimental effect than the assistance gained from the pictured arguments.

Table 11.3. Argument structure in single-word and sentence tests

	One argument	Two argument	Proportion correct
Single word	4/20 (0.20)	12/30 (0.40)	0.32
Sentence	12/24 (0.50)	11/29 (0.38)	0.43

A second sentence construction task, the TRIP (Whitworth, 1995b) was given to check sentence construction using one-, two- and three-argument structures. The TRIP has been devised to 'investigate word retrieval within sentences where nouns assume a thematic role in relation to the verb and overall sentence meaning' (Whitworth,1995a: 386). Sentences are used with increasing number of arguments thus affording the clinician a short, controlled task for investigating noun and verb retrieval in different sentence 'frames'. The test is divided into sections each of which require the same procedure. The tester first shows the stimulus pictures one by one, giving the correct target response. Each section is then re-presented, picture by picture, and the patient is required to give the target response. The first section elicits single words which subsequently appear in the sentence tasks: this is followed by sections containing sentences with one, two and three verb arguments.

LE was able to name all the pictures and scored 6/7 for the first section which comprised sentences containing one-argument verbs; 0/10 for the second section, sentences with two-argument verbs; and 1/5 for sentences with three-argument verbs in the last section. Although the amount of data is small, it would seem that LE found sentences with one-verb argument easier to produce than those requiring two or three. This is in line with the result obtained from the VECTA test and the predictions we made considering the results obtained by Zurif et al.

Errors in the sentence test

During all the production tasks LE frequently asked for feedback and queried whether her responses were correct. Her responses for the sentence construction test showed that most errors occurred as she failed to either access any verb (*this man is ...*) or accessed the incorrect verb (for example shown a picture of a man bricklaying her response was *this man is climbing ... no ... walling*). We can recall that LE's introspection on her performance on the sentence comprehension task suggested some occasional semantic confusion (for example she had difficulty deciding the target picture for the sentence which included *pull* vs. *push*). So we could speculate that there is a similar explanation for her production errors namely that she had access to the correct semantic area but difficulty in selecting or activating the precise lexical item. An alternative explanation for the errors on the single-word and sentence tests could be that having completed an unsuccessful lexical search, she then selected a semantically related verb even though she was aware that the word did not match the target: going for the best candidate available. She used her limited resources as best as she could, much as a L2 speaker might do. When unable to self-correct, she looked for reassurance and needed to be encouraged to continue with the task suggesting that as least on some level she was aware of her difficulties.

Spontaneous speech analyses

Text Unit analysis

Three samples of speech were analysed in order to gain information about her ability to use verbs in connected speech and to gain some information about the impact verb retrieval had on her ability to use grammatical structures. Three different samples of spontaneous speech were analysed, a description of her Easter bank holiday weekend; the retelling of the Cinderella story; and a description of a story depicted by a series of cartoons portraying a story about an ill-fated dinner party. The speech samples were segmented and tagged using Text Units (TUs) as the unit of analysis. Under this system, all speech is included for analysis except immediate and exact repetitions. The procedure used was one developed on the Reading Aphasia Project (Edwards, Garman and Knott, 1993; Edwards and Knott, 1994; and other publications). For the purpose of these analyses, seven types of TUs were logged: clauses, main and subordinate; multi-word utterances tagged as phrasal; single words tagged as lexical; minor, which included greetings, expletives, stereotypic phrases; unanalysed which included incomplete and unintelligible utterances.

The Weekend sample contained 100 TUs: the other two samples which consisted of 75 TUs (Cinderella) and 59 (Dinner Party), are expressed as proportions of 100. The distribution of TUs is displayed in Table 11.4. Values for a group of ten control subjects taken from Edwards and Bastiaanse (1998) are given in Table 11.5. As the age range of the control subjects was wide, a new set of control data was collected from a subject with a closer age match (25 compared with 29 years). The control subject was a post-graduate student and therefore had been in full-time education slightly longer than LE who would have graduated from nursing after approximately 16 years of education. Both subjects had been educated in Scotland. The new control data comprise three separate samples corresponding to the three samples collected from LE. Both sets of control data are given in Table 11.5.

Table 11.4. Distribution of LE's Text Units in three samples: proportional values

Text Units	Weekend	Cinderella	Dinner Party
Main clauses error free	32	49	37
Main clauses with errors	6	10.6	10
Subordinate clauses	10	12	3**
Phrasal	10	5*	13
Lexical	8	0	8
Minor	10*	2.6	3
Unanalysed	24*	18.6*	25*

* Outside normal range for controls.
** Outside normal range for controls and containing errors.

Table 11.5. Range for normal speakers ($n = 10$)

	Main clauses	Sub. clauses	Phrasal	Lexical	Minor	Unanalysed
	30–48	10–29	6–26	3–9	3–21	1–7

Values for one normal control matched for age, gender and education

Weekend	52	13	23	2	8	2
Cinderella	52	24	14	4	6	0
Dinner Party	55	7	27	1	8	2

It can be noted that the values obtained from the control group reveal considerable individual variation. By marking the proportions of LE's data that fall outside the range of the group rather than marking those categories which differ from the values obtained from the subject matched for age and education, we are taking a conservative approach to the analyses. A considerable proportion of the text, approximately a quarter in two of the samples, consisted of TUs which were either incomplete or contained errors which prevented analysis. However it can be seen that, despite considerable problems with output, she was able to create clauses including some subordinate clauses.

These results indicate that, notwithstanding a marked verb deficit, LE was reasonably successful at clause construction. The different values across the three samples suggest that, in some way, familiarity of content aided her production, at least in terms of clause production. The Cinderella sample (retelling a well-known story) contained the highest proportion of main clauses and the lowest proportion (19%) of unanalysed TUs: see Table 11.4. There was little difference in the proportion of either main clauses or unanalysed TUs produced in the other two samples suggesting that the presence of pictures did not enhance LE's ability to produce grammatically well-formed structures. Although the values for the three samples fall within the range obtained for the group of normal controls, the proportions for two of the samples, the Weekend and Dinner Party, are lower than those obtained for the subject matched for age and educational background.

Type–token ratio of verbs

The type–token ratios (ttrs) of lexical verbs in these samples were calculated to give a rather crude index of verb diversity. (Ratios were obtained by dividing the number of different lexical verb types by the number of verb tokens where *go think like* are types of lexical verbs: *go goes went* as well as repetitions of *go* are tokens of the lexical verb *go* and *thinks thought* as well as repetitions of *think* are tokens of *think* and so on. This rather crude measure gives an indication of the range of different types of lexical verbs used.) For this analysis, 250-word samples were taken from the samples used for the TU analysis. This sample is slightly smaller than that used by Edwards and Bastiaanse (1998) but, as in that paper, counts were based on total number of words except immediate and exact repetitions. Results are displayed in Table 11.6.

Table 11.6. Type–token ratios (ttr) of verbs

	Weekend	Cinderella	Dinner Party
Values for LE			
Types	15	16	10
Tokens	30	35	14
ttr	0.50	0.46	0.71
Values for age-matched control			
Types	16	23	23
Tokens	28	29	29
ttr	0.57	0.79	0.79

The Weekend sample which was unrehearsed, may be regarded as more representative of her everyday speech than the other two samples. In the Weekend sample the number of different types of lexical verbs was 15, the number of tokens 30 giving a ttr of 0.50. Bastiaanse, Edwards and Kiss (1996) report the range of ttrs for ten English controls being between 0.53 and 0.79 but averaging in the low 70s. Compared with these groups of data, LE would seem to be operating with a more restricted range of verbs although the number of verb *tokens* produced is sufficient to enable her to produce a proportion of clauses within the normal range. However, when compared with her age matched control we see that the values for LE are not so different.

In contrast, the ttr for the Cinderella Story, a more constrained task than that of recounting weekend activities, contained a relatively high proportion of clauses, including subordinate clauses but had the lowest ttr for verbs, (0.46). Contrasting these two samples, a story retell task and an unrestrained monologue, it might seem that the familiarity of the story aided the speaker in terms of using grammatical structures but this was achieved at the expense of verb diversity or at least in association with reduced lexical diversity. We can note that the values for the matched control are within the range of the control group. Unlike LE, the control subject produced a wider range of lexical verbs in this sample.

For the third text, the speaker was required to construct a novel story to describe a series of pictures, a more constrained task than either of the other two. In this task, LE produced a proportion of main clauses and a ttr for verbs which were within normal limits (0.71). However, in this sample, the proportion of subordinate clauses is low (in common with all three samples, the proportion of unanalysable TUs is high). A relatively high diversity of lexical verbs but a reduced proportion of sentence complexity is in line with the observations of Berndt, Mitchum, Haendinges and Sanderson (1997b) who observed a correlation between verb production and measures of sentence elaboration. Although it is important to be cautious in interpreting these data, it would appear that although the impaired lexical accessing skills and the syntactic skills interact, the nature of the task also has an effect. It seems that the pictures may have assisted lexical retrieval for LE, at least as measured by ttr, whilst having no influence on clause production. Not surprisingly, there was no similar effect seen for the normal control. For her, both constrained story-telling tasks resulted in a wider range of lexical verbs than the unrestrained retelling of her weekend activities.

Clauses and ttrs

If proportion of main clause TUs, proportion of subordinate clause TUs and ttr of verbs are taken as indices of syntactic and lexical production, then LE's performance is different for each of the three narrative tasks. The highest proportion of clause construction was observed in the Cinderella sample but it was in this sample that there was the most restricted range of lexical verbs. Retelling the events of her bank holiday weekend resulted in normal proportions of both types of clause TUs but, as in the Cinderella sample, a low ttr for verbs. In the Dinner Party sample, where there was pictorial support, a different picture emerged. LE managed a high proportion of main clauses and a normal ttr for verbs but this time the proportion of subordinate clauses was low.

These features are displayed in Table 11.7. Although each sample contains abnormal proportions of unanalysed TUs, other features which reflect the aphasia, vary between the samples.

Table 11.7. Clauses and lexical diversity of verbs

	Weekend	Cinderella	Dinner Party
Unanalysed Text Units	High	High	High
Main clauses	Normal	Normal	Normal
Sub. clauses	Normal	Normal	Low
Type–token ratio of verbs	Low	Low	Normal

The category of unanalysed TUs can be put aside because it is abnormally high (compared with all normal controls) for each sample. The category of main clause can be temporarily disregarded, this time because each sample contains proportions within the range of the normal controls. The two remaining categories of subordinate clauses and ttr give a crude index of syntactic complexity and lexical diversity. In the two tasks without any pictorial support the subject produced a proportion of subordinate clauses which fell within the normal range but the ratio of different lexical verbs to total number of verbs used was low. Like Berndt et al.'s five subjects who were able to produce sentences although dependent on 'light verbs', LE achieved a proportion of subordinate clauses within the normal range but at the cost of verb diversity. The reverse picture was found in the task where there was pictorial support. Here the ratio of different types to number of tokens of verbs used was within the normal range but the proportion of subordinate clauses was low compared with normal speakers. By comparing samples of spontaneous speech collected under three different conditions we can see how procedure might influence output in connected speech as well as the test conditions. The results suggest that different processing demands of the various tasks may impact differently on lexical and syntactic abilities in one patient as well as across patients (Edwards and Bastiaanse, 1998).

Verbs and their arguments

Results from the sentence construction tests support the notion that verbs taking two or three arguments are harder for agrammatic speakers to produce than those taking one argument. In the VECTA 50% of the verbs produced in sentences were one-place verbs and only 38% were two-place verbs. In the TRIP she was able to produce six out of the seven target sentences with one-place verbs but none of the target sentences with two-place verbs and only one of the five sentences with three-place verbs. However, when we examined her spontaneous connected speech there was no evidence that LE *only* had access to one argument verbs or that LE was using any kind of *strategy* in her spontaneous speech to use one-place verbs rather than two-place verbs. The distribution of verbs found in her spontaneous speech reflected the pattern found for both normal speakers and fluent aphasic speakers (Thompson, Shapiro, Li and Schendel, 1995;

Bastiaanse, Ewards and Kiss, 1996) although there are important variations between samples as shown in Table 11.8. It can be seen that in line
with Thompson et al.'s results, LE used both one-place and two-place
verbs frequently and, in line with normal speakers, two-place verbs were
more frequent than one-place verbs. It is true that she rarely used verbs
taking three arguments but these did occur as did verbs taking sentential
arguments although these values need to be viewed with caution. One of
the four logged in the Weekend sample and seven of the Cinderella
sample were *said*. She did use *where, when, who* and *that* but infre-
quently. Although there are different rates of opportunities for verbs
associated with one-, two- or three-place arguments, there are more two-
and indeed three-place argument verbs present than we might expect,
given the results from the TRIP test. The types of verbs produced in the
test conditions suggested a more limited access to verbs than was seen in
her spontaneous speech.

Table 11.8. Verbs and their arguments in spontaneous speech (proportions)

	Weekend		Cinderella		Dinner Party	
One-argument	4	(0.2)	8	(0.2)	3	(0.2)
Two-argument	19	(0.7)	19	(0.5)	10	(0.7)
Three-argument	0	(0.0)	1	(0.3)	2	(0.1)
S^i	4	(0.2)	8	(0.2)	0	(0.0)

Lexical errors in the spontaneous speech samples

The low ttr in two of the samples, the high number of unanalysed TUs in
all three samples and the variety of lexical errors she made, evidence the
reduced ability to retrieve a range of words. The comprehension tests had
demonstrated that she had, at some level, good representation of lexical
verbs but all production tasks showed that she had difficulty in accessing
them. Failure to access a lexical item and lexical errors (paraphasic errors)
contributed to the proportion of TUs logged as Main Clause with Errors:
see Table 11.4. A second type of error was with verb inflection but these
were less frequent. Clauses where verb inflection errors occurred were
also logged under Main clause with error. Examples of errors in main
clauses are given in Table 11.9.

When she failed to access a verb, there were several possible results: a
word with similar meaning might be used as in *throwing* for *batting* and
for *heading*; the lexical verb might be omitted, for example, *because they
said they didn't (unintelligible) on poor Cinders*; a non-specific verb
might be used, for example, *and they get all around to do (this) this
slipper thing*; the sentence might be abandoned as in the first two
attempts here, *so when they – – two three – – when they're all – when
they're all done*. Omission of a verb and abandonment of an utterance

diminished her communicative competence as did resorting to non-specific verbs such as *do*, and the use of a semantically related verb was only occasionally successful and observed mainly in the test conditions rather than in the free narratives. Although LE did produce a reasonable account of her weekend, the story of Cinderella and produced a story to fit the series of cartoons, these were difficult tasks for her.

Table 11.9. Errors in main clauses

Omissions:	*they didn't on poor Cinders*
	and poor old Cinders was terribly
	and they happily ever after
Paraphasic errors	*so there's this man and his three /sizez/*
Inflectional errors	*so he (get) get a few men*
	and other people be so

Discussion and summary

Tests confirmed that retrieval of lexical items remained a problem for LE and this impairment was especially marked for verbs. The reduced ability to access verbs in continuous speech contributed to her difficulty in constructing grammatical sequences which was apparent in the high proportion of unanalysed TUs in all spontaneous speech samples. However, difficulty with retrieving verbs could not account for a reduction of subordinate clauses in the Dinner Party sample. If she was able to retrieve sufficient verbs to form a proportion of main clauses which falls within normal limits, then a verb deficit is not a sufficient explanation. Baastiaanse and Edwards (1998) have argued that a reduction in subordinate clauses signifies a reduction in ability to use complex grammatical constructions. Such a finding would be less surprising in this patient, LE, who had been diagnosed as agrammatic, than in the fluent aphasic patients reported on by Bastiaanse and Edwards. As with the findings for the fluent aphasic speakers, LE's three spontaneous speech samples demonstrated dissociations between grammatical complexity and verb diversity. In the Dinner Party sample there was evidence of reduced grammatical complexity yet the widest range of lexical verbs. The other two samples showed the reverse pattern: here she had enough control over grammatical construction to use both main and subordinate clauses but at the expense of the range of lexical verbs she used elsewhere.

This is not to suggest that she had conscious strategies at her disposal but to suggest that these dissociations illustrate the interdependency of lexical and syntactic skills. In very simple terms, if resources are limited there may be a trade-off between lexical retrieval and the use of grammatically complex structures. Efforts to increase the range of verbs (as seemed to be the case when she needed to create a text to match a series of pictures) was at the expense of subordination, syntactic complexity. In the tasks where she had more control of the text produced, she produced normal proportions of both main and subordinate clauses but only by using a limited range of lexical verbs. In these samples she was either able to produce a normal proportion of subordinate clauses or a range of ttrs of verbs within normal limits.

Traditional descriptions of Broca's aphasia include terms such as 'effortful speech' or 'slow speech'. It has also been noted above that the subjects with Broca's aphasia were slower in their responses than the normal controls on the cross-modality lexical decision tasks (Shapiro, Zurif and Grimshaw, 1987). As predicted, LE was very slow on all tasks given in this assessment. She was cautious in her responses, pausing between items or utterances and looking for reassurance. She either did not have the ability to make quick internal checks on the accuracy of her output or she did not have confidence in her own linguistic judgments. The slow reaction times would seem to be another indicator of the stressed system and limited resources.

Testing produced conflicting results. Testing of sentence construction indicated that, in line with our initial predictions based on the research of Shapiro and colleagues, LE had considerably more difficulty constructing sentences when the verb of the sentence was associated with two or more arguments. This would seem to support the claims made about the clinical performance of agrammatic speakers (Byng, 1988) and the need to investigate this difficulty (Whitworth, 1996). Contrary to those findings, however, this preference was not found in the single-word tests and, more importantly, there was no clear evidence in her spontaneous speech that verb retrieval was affected by associated argument structure. The results of the analyses of her spontaneous speech revealed that although diversity of lexical verbs was reduced (at least in two of the samples), she was able to use verbs associated with one, two and sentential arguments and there were no major differences across the three samples. Speech production outside the constraints of the test format improved her recall of transitive verbs. The requirements of sentential structure within connected speech aided the production of verbs and their associated arguments. Although she performed poorly on the sentences in the TRIP there was no evidence in her spontaneous speech that difficulty with verb retrieval was associated with the number of arguments associated with the verb. As Shapiro and colleagues found, if she retrieved a verb she had full access to the associated arguments.

Distressingly for LE, however, she did not have ready access to all verbs. Although the distribution of verbs in her spontaneous speech, classified by the number of associated arguments, resembled that of normal speakers, the diversity of lexical verbs was restricted in two of the three speech samples. In the third sample which was elicited by asking LE to describe a series of cartoon pictures, the ttr (the metric used in this study for verb diversity) for verbs was within normal limits. Was it the case, then, that the presence of pictures aided verb production? It is not possible to confirm this from the current test results: tests requiring production of a single verb without picture stimuli (such as those used by Berndt et al.) might help to unravel these factors. In fact Berndt and colleagues found that four of their subjects who had greater difficulty retrieving verbs than nouns did perform better on tasks where picture stimuli were used. If this is the case for LE, then maybe visual information boots the lexical representation and aids retrieval.

These results revealed that LE's problem was with the semantic representation and production of some verbs. Whereas semantic representation did interfere with access, and this is seen most clearly in the errors made in the action naming test, the number of associated argument structures appeared not to exert much effect. Once LE had to produce a verb within a sentential structure, in tasks where she was required to convey a story or events, the effect of argument structure was lost, at least for the one-argument and two-argument verbs. For this patient, although sensitivity to argument structure could be demonstrated in some tests, her reduced retrieval of a range of different lexical verbs had a more profound effect on her spontaneous speech. If she does have some semantic representation of verbs and, as claimed above, full representation of associated argument structures then this would indeed promote sentence construction.

Verb deficits are not straightforward and this case highlights the clinical necessity of exploring verb production in a number of different ways. As has been demonstrated, if clinical decisions are based on data from only single-word tests, or only sentence tests, then the clinician may be gaining skewed information. Although such tests *may* throw light on certain aspects of language production, they do not necessarily reflect the patient's ability in connected speech. Furthermore, the potential complexity of a verb deficit underlines the hazards of using simple, short tests as base lines which are to be used either to motivate therapy or to judge the efficacy of therapy. The results reported here demonstrate the need to use a variety of testing procedures, including the analysis of speech samples. Although testing is time consuming, the breadth of information gained from a range of test procedures is likely to compensate for the time spent.

Despite having worked on a neuro-surgical ward for several years, a ward on which there were often patients with aphasia, LE said that she had never thought about either the nature or the effect of aphasia. Although distressed by her performances, she was keen to participate in the testing and very interested to learn more about her language deficits. Testing demonstrated to her as well as to her clinicians that although she had difficulty accessing verbs she had almost normal representation of verbs: she could understand most, although not all verbs. There were very varied results from the tests of production. Tests of single verb production and tests of verb production within sentences revealed a verb-retrieval deficit. The analyses of the spontaneous speech samples demonstrated that there was little evidence to support the notion that the number of arguments associated with a verb-affected verb retrieval despite the results on the TRIP. However, verb retrieval did seem to be compromised when the system was generating complex grammar.

It is clearly desirable for clinicians to initiate theoretically motivated practice. But before therapy can start, it is important for the clinician to conduct a comprehensive assessment even though the relationship between linguistic assessment and therapeutic procedures is not a straightforward matter (Edwards and Garman, 1989). Ten years on from this observation, although our knowledge of aphasia has increased, the links remain difficult to forge. This small battery of tests reported here informed the therapist in a number of ways. Results confirmed the therapist's observation that the speaker did, indeed, have problems with verbs, helped reveal the weak influence of argument structure, demonstrated that performance on single-word tests did not predict language skills in connected speech and highlighted how connected speech might differ according to the elicitation method. Faced with this array of results, it would be difficult to see how any therapy which is to be effective can be promoted without first conducting a range of linguistically based tests. For this patient, the results gained from a range of tests gave no credence to working on 'simple' one-place verbs rather than verbs with two or more arguments nor did they suggest that single-word tasks might be more beneficial than encouraging verbs within sentential contexts. Practice in using a range of verbs in sentences within textually communicative contexts would appear to be the most helpful advice for this patient, advice which would have been in direct contrast to that given had only one of the tests been given.

Acknowledgements

I would like to thank Lindsey Hovarth for bringing LE to my attention and sharing her clinical observations with me. I would also like to thank Judith Rispens for her translation of the VECTA test and Richard Ingham and David Lightfoot for their comments on this chapter.

References

Abney S (1987) The English noun phrase in its sentential aspects. Unpublished doctoral dissertation, Massachusetts Institute of Technology, Cambridge.

Ahlsén E, Darvins C (1990) Agrammatism in Swedish: two case studies. In Menn L, Obler L (eds) Agrammatic Aphasia: A Cross-language Narrative Sourcebook. Philadelphia, John Benjamin's Publishing Company.

Alexander M, Naeser MA, Palumbo CL (1990) Broca's area aphasias: aphasia after lesions including the frontal operculum. Neurology 40: 353–62.

Antal L (1977) Egy új magyar nyelvtan felé (Towards a new Hungarian grammar). Budapest: Magvetô Kiadó.

Armon-Lotem S (1996) A parametric approach to functional heads and the acquisition of Hebrew. PhD dissertation, Tel Aviv University.

Avrutin S (in press) Comprehension of discourse-linked and non-discourse-linked questions by children and Broca's aphasics. In Grodzinsky Y, Shapiro LP, Swinney D (eds) Language and the Brain: Representation and Processing. San Diego: Academic Press.

Badecker W, Caramazza A (1985a) On considerations of method and theory governing the use of clinical categories in neurolinguistics and cognitive neuropsychology: the case against agrammatism. Cognition 20: 97–125.

Badecker W, Caramazza A (1985b) A final brief in the case against agrammatism: The role of theory in the selection of data. Cognition 24, 277–82.

Baker M, Johnson K, Roberts I (1989) Passive arguments raised. Linguistic Inquiry 20: 219–51.

Barrs A, Lasnik H (1986) A note on anaphora and double objects. Linguistic Inquiry 17: 347–54.

Basso A, Razzano C, Faglioni P, Zanobio ME (1990) Confrontation naming, picture description and action naming in aphasic patients. Aphasiology 4: 185–95.

Bastiaanse R (1991) Naming of instrumental verbs in aphasia: an explorative study. Clinical Linguistics and Phonetics 5: 355–68.

Bastiaanse R (1995) Broca's aphasia: a syntactic and/or morphological disorder? a case study. Brain and Language 48: 1–32.

Bastiaanse R, Jonkers R (1998) Verb retrieval in action naming and spontaneous speech in agrammatic and anomic aphasia. Aphasiology 12(11): 951–69.

Bastiaanse R, Van Zonneveld R (1998) On the relation between verb inflection and verb position in Dutch agrammatic aphasics. Brain and Language 64: 165–81.

Bastiaanse R, Jonkers R, Moltmaker-Osinga U (1995) Aspects of lexical verbs in the spontaneous speech of agrammatic and anomic patients. In Jonkers R, Kaan E, Wiegel A (eds) Language and Cognition 5. Groningen: University of Groningen.

Bastiaanse R, Edwards S, Kiss K (1996) Fluent aphasia in three languages: aspects of spontaneous speech. Aphasiology 10(6): 561–75.

Bates E, Friederici A, Wulfeck B (1987) Grammatical morphology in aphasia: evidence from three languages. Cortex 23: 545–74.

Bates E, MacWhinney B (1987) Competition, variation, and language learning. In MacWhinney B (ed) Mechanisms of Language Acquisition. New Jersey: Lawrence Erlbaum Associates.

Bates E, Wulfeck B (1989) Comparative aphasiology: a cross-linguistic approach to language breakdown. Aphasiology 3: 111–42.

Benedet MJ, Christiansen JA, Goodglass H (1998) A cross-linguistic study of grammatical morphology in Spanish- and English-speaking agrammatic patients. Cortex 34: 309–36.

Berman RA, Armon-Lotem S (1996) How grammatical are early verbs? Les annals littéraires de l'université de Besancon.

Berndt RS, Mitchum CC, Haendiges AN, Sanderson J (1997a) Verb retrieval in aphasia 1: Characterizating Single Word Impairments. Brain and Language 56: 68–106.

Berndt RS, Mitchum CC, Haendiges AN, Sanderson J (1997b) Verb retrieval in aphasia: 2. Relationship to sentence processing. Brain and Language 56: 107–37.

Bever TG and McElree B (1988) Empty categories access their antecedents during comprehension. Linguistic Inquiry 19: 35–44.

Bickerton D (1981) Roots of Language. Ann Arbor, MI: Karona.

Boland J (1996) The relationship between syntactic and semantic processes in sentence comprehension. Department of Psychology, Ohio State University. Unpublished manuscript

Bradley DC, Garrett MF, Zurif EB (1980) Syntactic deficits in Broca's aphasia. In Caplan D (ed) Biological Studies of Mental Processes. Cambridge, MA: MIT Press.

Breedin S, Martin R (1996) Patterns of verb impairment in aphasia: an analysis of four cases. Cognitive Neuropsychology 13: 51–91.

Bresnan J, Kanerva JM (1989) The thematic hierarchy and locative inversion in UG. Semantics 6: Syntax and the Lexicon. San Diego, CA: Academic Press.

Brody M (1990) Remarks on the order of elements in the Hungarian focus field. In Kenesei I (ed) Approaches to Hungarian 3. Szeged: József Attila Tudományegyetem.

Brookshire RH, Nicholas LE (1994) Speech sample size and test–retest stability of connected speech measures for adults with aphasia. Journal of Speech and Hearing Research 37: 399–407.

Burnage G (1990) A Guide for Users. Nijmegen: CELEX Centre for Lexical Information.

Byng S (1988) Sentence processing deficits: theory and therapy. Cognitive Neuropsychology 5: 629–76.

Byng S, Black M (1989) Some aspects of sentence production in aphasia. Aphasiology 3: 241–63.

Canseco-Gonzalez E, Shapiro LP, Zurif EB, Baker E (1990) Predicate-argument structure as a link between linguistic and nonlinguistic representations. Brain and Language 39: 391–404.

Caplan D (1986) In defense of agrammatism Cognition 24: 263–76.

Caplan D (1991) Agrammatism is a theoretically coherent aphasia category. Brain and Language 40: 274–81.

Caplan D, Futter C (1986) Assignment of thematic roles to nouns in sentence comprehension by an agrammatic patient. Brain and Language 27: 117–34.

Caplan D, Hildebrandt N (1988) Disorders of Syntactic Comprehension. Cambridge, MA: MIT Press.

Caplan D, Alpert N, Waters G (1998) Effects of syntactic structure and propositional number on patterns of rCBF. Journal of Cognitive Neuroscience 10: 541–52.

Caramazza AE, Zurif EB (1976) Dissociation of algorithmic and heuristic processes in language comprehension: evidence from aphasia. Brain and Language 3: 572–82.

Caramazza AE, Miceli G (1991) Selective impairment of thematic role assignment in sentence processing. Brain and Language 41: 402–36.

Caramazza AE, Grober C, Garvey, Yates J (1977) Comprehension of anaphoric pronouns. Journal of Verbal Learning and Verbal Behavior 16: 601–9.

Chen S, Bates E (1998) The dissociation between nouns and verbs in Broca's and Wernicke's aphasia: findings from Chinese. Aphasiology 12: 5–36.

Chierchia G (1984) Topics in the syntax and semantics of infinitives and gerunds. PhD dissertation, University of Massachusetts, Amherst, MA.

Chomsky N (1957) Syntactic Structures. The Hague: Mouton.

Chomsky N (1965) Aspects of a Theory of Syntax. Cambridge, MA: MIT Press.

Chomsky N (1973) Conditions of transformations. In Anderson SR, Kiparsy P (eds) A Festschrift for Morris Halle. New York: Holt & Reinhardt.

Chomsky N (1981) Lectures on Government and Binding: The Pisa Lectures. Dordrecht: Foris.

Chomsky, N (1986a) Barriers. Cambridge, MA: MIT Press.

Chomsky N (1986b) Knowledge of Language. New York: Praeger.

Chomsky, N (1992) A minimalist program for linguistic theory. MIT Occasional Papers in Linguistics 1. Cambridge, MA: MIT.

Chomsky N (1993) A minimalist program for linguistic theory. In Hale K, Keyser J (eds) The View from Building 20. Cambridge, MA: MIT Press, pp. 1–52.

Chomsky N (1995) The Minimalist Program. Cambridge, MA: MIT Press.

Cinque G (1990) Types of A-bar Dependencies. Cambridge, MA: MIT Press.

Coltheart M, Patterson K, Marshall JC (eds) (1980) Deep Dyslexia. London: Routledge & Kegan Paul.

Corbett AT, Chang FR (1983) Pronoun disambiguation: accessing potential antecedents. Memory and Cognition 11: 283–94.

Crain S, Fodor J (1985) How can grammars help parsers? In Dowty DR, Karttunen L, Zwicky AM (eds) Natural Language Parsing. Cambridge: Cambridge University Press.

Crain S, McKee C (1985) Acquisition of structural restrictions on anaphora. In Proceedings of the Sixteenth Annual Meeting, NELS, GLSA, University of Massachusetts at Amherst.

Dalrymple M (1991) Against reconstruction in ellipsis. Technical report No. SSL-91-114. Xerox.

Davidoff J, Masterson J (1996) The development of picture naming: differences between verbs and nouns. Journal of Neurolinguistics 9: 69–83.

De Bleser R, Bayer J (1990) Morphological reading errors in a German case of deep dyslexia. In Nespoulous, JL, Villiard P (eds) Morphology, Phonology, and Aphasia. New York: Springer

De Bleser R, Luzzatti C (1994) Morphological processing in Italian agrammatic speakers syntactic implementation of inflectional morphology. Brain and Language 46: 21–40.

De Vincenzi M (1996) Syntactic analysis in sentence comprehension: effects of dependency types and grammatical constraints. Journal of Psycholinguistic Research 25: 117–33.

Dowty DR (1991) Thematic proto-roles and argument selection. Language 67: 547–619

Dromi E, Leonard LB, Shteiman M (1993) The grammatical morphology of Hebrew-speaking children with specific language impairment: some competing hypotheses. Journal of Speech and Hearing Research 36: 760–71.

Dronkers N, Wilkin D, Van Valin R, Redfern B, Jaeger J (1994) A reconsideration of the brain areas involved in the disruption of morpho-syntactic comprehension. Brain and Language 47: 461–3.

Edwards S, Garman M (1989) Case study of a fluent aphasic: the relation between linguistic assessment and therapeutic intervention. In Grunwell P, James A (eds) The Functional Evaluation of Language Disorders. London: Croom Helm, pp. 163–87.

Edwards S, Knott R (1994) Assessing spontaneous language abilities of aphasic speakers. Language Testing 11: 49–64.

Edwards S, Bastiaanse R (1998) Diversity in the lexical and syntactic abilities of fluent aphasic speakers. Aphasiology 12: 99–117.

Edwards S, Garman M, Knott R (1993) Short report: the grammatical characterization of aphasic language. Aphasiology 7: 217–20.

Fillmore CJ (1988) The mechanisms of 'construction grammar'. Proceedings of the 14th Annual Meeting of the Berkeley Linguistics Society, University of California, Berkeley.

Fodor JD (1989) Empty categories in sentence processing. Special Issue: Parsing and Interpretation. Language and Cognitive Processes 4 (3-4, SI155-SI209).

Fox D, Grodzinsky Y (1998) Children's passive: a view from the by-phrase. Linguistic Inquiry 29: 311–32.

Francis WN, Kucera H (1982) Frequency Analysis of English Usage: Lexicon and Grammar. Boston, MA: Houghton Mifflin.

Frazier L (1978) On comprehending sentences: syntactic parsing strategies. Unpublished doctoral dissertation, University of Connecticut, Storrs.

Frazier L, Clifton C (1995) Construal. Cambridge, MA: MIT Press.

Frazier L, McNamara P (1995) Favor referential representation. Brain and Language 49: 224–40.

Frazier L, Flores d'Arcais GB (1989) Filler-driven parsing: a study of gap-filling in Dutch. Journal of Memory and Language 28: 331–44.

Friedmann N (1994) Morphology in agrammatism: a dissociation between tense and agreement. MA thesis, Tel Aviv University.

Friedmann N (1998) Functional categories in agrammatic production: a cross linguistic study. Doctoral dissertation, Tel Aviv University.

Friedmann N, Grodzinsky Y (1997) Tense and agreement in agrammatic production: pruning the syntactic tree. Brain and Language 56: 397–425.

Garman M (1990) Psycholinguistics. Cambridge: Cambridge University Press.

Garnsey SM, Tanenhaus MK, Chapman RM (1989) Evoked potentials and the study of sentence comprehension. Journal of Psycholinguistic Research 18(1): 51–60.

Gazdar G, Klein E, Pullum GK, Sag L (1985) Generalized Phrase Structure Grammar. Cambridge, MA: Harvard University Press.

Gerratt B, Jones D (1987) Aphasic performance on a lexical decision task: multiple meanings and word frequency. Brain and Language 30, 106–15.

Goldberg AE (1995) A Construction Grammar Approach to Argument Structure. Chicago: The University of Chicago Press.

Goodglass H (1993) Understanding Aphasia. San Diego: Academic Press.

Goodglass H, Mayer J (1958) Agrammatism in aphasia. Journal of Speech and Hearing Disorders 23: 99–111.

Goodglass H, Kaplan E (1972) The Assessment of Aphasia and Related Disorders. Philadelphia: Lea and Febiger.

Goodglass H, Geschwind N (1976) Language disorders (aphasia). In Carterette EC, Friedman MP (eds) Handbook of Perception 7. New York: Academic Press.

Goodglass H, Gleason JB, Bernholtz NA, Hyde MR (1972) Some linguistic structures in the speech of Broca's aphasia. Cortex 8: 191–212.

Gottfried M, Menn L, Holland A (1997) Verb argument-structure and aphasic repetition. Brain and Language 60: 36–8.

Graetz P, Bleser R De, Willmes K (1992) Akense Afasietest. Lisse: Swets and Zeitlinger.

Grimshaw J (1979) Complement selection and the lexicon. Linguistic Inquiry 10: 279–326.

Grimshaw J (1987) Unaccusatives: an overview. In McDonough J, Plunkett B (eds) Proceedings of NELS 17, 1986, Volume 1, GLSA, University of Massachusetts, Amherst, MA, pp. 244–58.

Grimshaw J (1990) Argument Structure. Cambridge, MA: MIT Press.

Grodzinsky Y (1986) Language deficits and the theory of syntax. Brain and Language 27: 135–59.

Grodzinsky Y (1990) Theoretical Perspectives on Language Deficits. Cambridge, MA: MIT Press.

Grodzinsky Y (1991) There is an entity called agrammatism. Brain and Language 41: 555–64.

Grodzinsky Y (1995a) A restrictive theory of agrammatic comprehension. Brain and Language 50: 27–51.

Grodzinsky Y (1995b) Trace deletion, Theta-roles, and cognitive strategies. Brain and Language 51: 469–97.

Grodzinsky Y (in press) The neurology of syntax: language use without Broca's area. Behavioral and Brain Sciences.

Grodzinsky Y, Finkel L (1998) The neurology of empty categories: aphasics' failure to detect ungrammaticality. Journal of Cognitive Neuroscience 10: 281–92.

Haarmann HJ, Kolk HHJ (1991) A computer model of the temporal course of agrammatic sentence understanding: the effects of variation in severity and sentence complexity. Cognitive Science 25: 49–87.

Haarmann HJ, Kolk HHJ (1994) On-line sensitivity to subject-verb agreement violations in Broca's aphasics: the role of syntactic complexity and time. Brain and Language 46, 493–516.

Hackl M (1995) Verb-Zweit bei Agrammatismus: Zwei Fallstudien. MA dissertation, Universitat Wien.

Haegeman L (1992) Introduction to Government and Binding Theory. Oxford: Blackwell.

Haegeman L (1995) The Syntax of Negation. Cambridge: Cambridge University Press.

Hagiwara H (1995) The breakdown of functional categories and the economy of derivation. Brain and Language 50: 92–116.

Hagiwara H, Caplan D (1990) Syntactic comprehension in Japanese aphasics: effects of category and thematic role order. Brain and Language 38: 159–70.

Heeschen C (1985) Agrammatism versus paragrammatism: a fictitious opposition In: Kean MI (ed) Agrammatism. New York: Academic Press.

Hickok G (1993) Parallel parsing: evidence from re-activation in garden path sentences. Journal of Psycholinguistic Research 22: 239–50.

Hickok G, Avrutin S (1995) Representation, referentiality, and processing in agrammatic comprehension: two case studies. Brain and Language 50: 10–26.

Hickok G, Avrutin S (1996) Comprehension of Wh-questions by two agrammatic Broca's aphasics. Brain and Language 52: 314–27.

Hickok G, Zurif EB, Canseco-Gonzales E (1993) Structural description of agrammatic comprehension. Brain and Language 45: 371–95.

Horvath J (1986) Focus in the Theory of Grammar and the Syntax of Hungarian. Dordrecht: Foris.

Hyams N (1996) The underspecification of functional categories in early grammar. In Clahsen H (ed) Generative Perspectives on Language Acquisition. Philadelphia: John Benjamins, pp. 91–127.

Jackendoff R (1972) Semantic Interpretation in Generative Grammar. Cambridge, MA: MIT Press.

Jackendoff R (1987) The status of thematic relations in linguistic theory. Linguistic Inquiry 18: 369–411.

Jackendoff R (1990a) On Larson's treatment of the double object construction. Linguistic Inquiry 21: 427–55.

Jackendoff R (1990b) Semantic Structures. Cambridge, MA: MIT Press.

Jackendoff R (1997) The Architecture of the Language Faculty. Cambridge, MA: MIT Press.

Jaeggli O (1986) Passive. Linguistic Inquiry 17: 587–22.

Jastrzembski J (1981) Multiple meanings, number of related meanings, frequency of occurrence, and the lexicon. Cognitive Psychology 13: 278–305.

Jastrzembski J, Stanners R (1975) Multiple word meanings and lexical search speed. Journal of Verbal Learning and Verbal Behavior 14, 534–7.

Jones EV (1984) Word order processing in aphasia: effect of verb semantics. In Rose PC (ed) Advances in Neurology 42: Progress in Aphasiology. New York: Raven Press, pp. 159–81.

Jonkers, R (1998) Comprehension and production of verbs in aphasic speakers. Groninjen, Grodil (Groninjen dissertations in Linguistics) 25.

Jonkers R, Bastiaanse R (1994) Verb Elicitation and Comprehension Tasks for Aphasics. Department of Linguistics, University of Groningen, The Netherlands.

Jonkers R, Bastiaanse R (1996) The influence of instrumentality and transitivity on action naming in Broca's and anomic aphasia. Brain and Language 55: 37–9.

Kaplan E, Goodglass H, Weintraub S (1983) Boston Naming Test.Philadelphia: Lea & Febiger.

Kaplan R, Bresnan J (1982) Lexical-functional grammar: a formal system for grammatical representation. In Bresnan J (ed) The Mental Representation of Grammatical Relations. Cambridge, MA: MIT Press.

Kay J, Lesser R, Coltheart M (1992) Psycholinguistic Assessment of Language Processing in Aphasia. Hove: Erlbaum.

Kayne R (1984) Connectedness and binary branching. Dordrecht: Foris.

Kean ML (1977) The linguistic interpretation of aphasic syndromes. Cognition 5: 9–46.

Kehler A (1994) Common topics and coherent situations: interpreting ellipsis in the context of discourse inference. In Proceedings of the 32nd Conference of the Association of Computational Linguistics.

Kellas G, Ferraro FR, Simpson G (1988) Lexical ambiguity and the time-course of attentional allocation in word recognition. Journal of Experimental Psychology, Human Perception and Performance 14: 601–9.

Kiss KE (1998) Effect of verb complexity on agrammatic aphasics' sentence production. In Bastiaanse R, Grodzinsky Y (eds) Advances in the Neurolinguistic Study of Language. London: Whurr.

Kiss KE, Mészáros É, Kiefer F (1992) Processing of different types of verbs in Hungarian aphasics. Morphological and Phonological Disturbances in Aphasia, Abstracts (unpublished).

Kiss KE (1987) Configurationality in Hungarian. Studies in Natural Language and Linguistic Theory. Dordrecht: Reidel.

Kiss KE (1990) Against treating Hungarian as a V-second language. In Kenesei I (ed) Approaches to Hungarian 3. Szeged: József Attila Tudományegyetem.

Kiss KE (1994a) Sentence structure and word order. In Kiefer F and Kiss KE (eds) Syntax and Semantics: The Syntactic Structure of Hungarian 27. San Diego: Academic Press.

Kiss KE (1994b) Genericity, predication, and focus. In Bánréti Z (eds) Papers in the Theory of Grammar. Research Institute for Linguistics of Hungarian Academy of Sciences.

Kiss K (1995) NP movement, operator movement, and scrambling in Hungarian. In Kiss KE (ed) Discourse Configurational Languages. Oxford: Oxford University Press.

Klein E, Sag I (1985) Type-driven translation. Linguistics and Philosophy 8: 163–202.

Klein W, Perdue C (1998) The basic variety. Ms. Nijmegen, The Netherlands: Max-Planck-Institut für Psycholinguistik.

Kluender R (1998) On the distinction between strong and weak islands: a processing perspective. In Syntax and Semantics: The Limits of Syntax. San Diego: Academic Press.

Kohn SE, Lorch MP, Pearson DM (1989) Verb finding in aphasia. Cortex 25: 57–69.

Kolk H. (1995) A time-based approach to agrammatic production. Brain and Language 50: 282–303.

Kolk H, Heeschen C (1992) Agrammatism, paragrammatism and the management of language. Language and Cognitive Processes 7: 82–129.

Kolk H, Weijts M (1996) Judgments of semantic anomaly in agrammatic patients: argument movement, syntactic complexity, and the use of heuristics. Brain and Language 54: 86–136.

Kolk H, Van Grunsven M, Keyser M (1985) On parallelism between production and comprehension in agrammatism. In Kean ML (ed) Agrammatism. London: Academic Press.

Komlósy A (1994) Complements and adjuncts, syntax and semantics. In Kiefer F, Kiss K (eds) The Syntactic Structure of Hungarian 27. San Diego: Academic Press.

Koster J (1975) Dutch as an SOV language. Linguistic Analysis 1: 111–36.

Lapointe S (1985) A theory of verb form use in the speech of agrammatic aphasics. Brain and Language 24: 100–55.

Lapointe S, Dell GS (1989) A synthesis of some recent work in sentence production. In Carlson GN, Tanenhaus MK (eds) Linguistic Structure in Language Processing, Dordrecht: Reidel pp. 107–56.

Larson R (1988) On the double object construction. Linguistic Inquiry 19: 335–92.

Lebeaux D (1988) Language acquisition and the form of grammar. Unpublished doctoral dissertation, University of Massachusetts, Amherst.

Lee C (1990) Some hypotheses concerning the evolution of polysemous words. Journal of Psycholinguistic Research 4: 211–19.

Leonard LB (1995) Functional categories in the grammars of children with specific language impairment. Journal of Speech and Hearing Research 38: 1270–83.

Leonard LB, Loeb DF (1988) Government-binding theory and some of its applications: a tutorial. Journal of Speech and Hearing Research 31: 515–24.

Levin B (1993) English verb classes and alternations: a preliminary investigation. Chicago: University of Chicago Press.

Levin B, Rappaport-Hovav M (1995) The Unaccusative Hypothesis at the Syntax–Semantics Interface. Cambridge, MA: MIT Press.

Linebarger M (1989) Neuropsychological evidence for linguistic modularity. In Carlson G, Tanenhaus M (eds) Linguistic Structure in Language Processing. Dordrecht: Kluwer.

Linebarger M (1990) Neuropsychology of sentence parsing. In Caramazza A (ed)

Cognitive Neuropsychology and Neurolinguistics: Advances in Models of Cognitive Function and Impairment. Hillsdale, NJ: Erlbaum, pp. 55–122.

Linebarger M, Schwartz M, Saffran EM (1983) Sensitivity to grammatical structure in so-called agrammatic aphasics. Cognition 13: 361–92.

Lobeck A (1992) Licensing and identification of ellipted categories in English. In Berman S, Hestvik A (eds) (1992) Proceedings of the Stuttgart Ellipsis Workshop (Arbeitspapiere des Sonderforschungsbereich 340, Bericht Nr. 29). Heidelberg, IBM Germany.

Lonzi L, Luzzatti C (1993) Relevance of adverb distribution for the analysis of sentence representation in agrammatic patients. Brain and Language 45, 306–17.

Love T, Swinney D (1996) Co-reference processing and levels of analysis in object-relative constructions: demonstration of antecedent reactivation with the cross-modal priming paradigm. Journal of Psycholinguistic Research 25(1): 5–24.

McCarthy R, Warrington EK (1985) Category specificity in an agrammatic patient: the relative impairment of verb retrieval and comprehension. Neuropsychologia 23: 709–27.

MacDonald MC, Pearlmutter NJ, Seidenberg MS (1994) The lexical nature of syntactic ambiguity resolution. Psychological Review 101(4): 676–703.

McElree B, Griffith T (1995) Syntactic and thematic processing in sentence comprehension: evidence for a temporal dissociation. Journal of Experimental Psychology: Learning, Memory and Cognition 21: 134–57.

McKoon G, Ratcliff R (1994) Sentential context and on-line lexical decision. Journal of Experimental Psychology: Learning, Memory and Cognition 20(5): 1239–43.

McKoon G, Ratcliff R, Albritton D (1996) Sentential context effects on lexical decisions with a cross-modal instead of an all-visual procedure. Journal of Experimental Psychology 22(6): 1494–7

MacWhinney B, Osman-Sági J (1991) Inflectional marking in Hungarian aphasics. Brain and Language 4: 165–83.

Magnúsdóttir S, Thráinsson H (1990) Agrammatism in Icelandic: two case studies. In Menn L, Obler L (eds) Agrammatic Aphasia: A Cross-language Narrative Sourcebook. Philadelphia: John Benjamin's Publishing Company.

Manzini R (1983) On control and control theory. Linguistic Inquiry 14: 421–46.

Marácz L (1990) V movement in Hungarian: a case of minimality. In Kenesei I (ed) Approaches to Hungarian 3. Szeged: József Attila Tudományegyetem.

Marantz A (1995) The minimalist program. In Webelhuth G (ed) Government and Binding Theory and the Minimalist Program. Oxford: Basil Blackwell.

Marshall J, Pring T, Chiat S (1993) Sentence processing therapy: working at the level of the event. Aphasiology 7: 177–99.

Mauner G, Fromkin V, Cornell T (1993) Comprehension and acceptability judgments in agrammatism: disruption in the syntax of referential dependency. Brain and Language 45: 340–70.

Menn L (1990) Agrammatism in English: two case studies. In Menn L, Obler L (eds) Agrammatic Aphasia: A Cross-language Narrative Sourcebook. Philadelphia: John Benjamin's Publishing Company.

Menn L, Obler L (eds) (1990) Agrammatic Aphasia: A Cross-language Narrative Sourcebook. Philadelphia: John Benjamin's Publishing Company.

Meyer DE, Schvaneveldt RW, Ruddy MG (1975) Loci of contextual effects on visual word recognition. In Rabbit PMA, Dornic S (eds) Attention and Performance V. New York: Academic Press.

Miceli G, Caramazza A (1988) Dissociation of inflectional and derivational morphology. Brain and Language 35: 24–65.

Miceli G, Mazzucchi A (1990) Agrammatism in Italian: two case studies. In Menn L, Obler L (eds) Agrammatic Aphasia: A Cross-language Narrative Sourcebook. Philadelphia: John Benjamin's Publishing Company.

Miceli G, Mazzucchi A, Menn L, Goodglass H (1983) Contrasting cases of Italian agrammatic aphasia without comprehension disorder. Brain and Language 19: 65–97.

Miceli G, Silveri MC, Villa G, Caramazza A (1984) On the basis of the agrammatics' difficulty in producing main verbs. Cortex 20: 207–20.

Miceli G, Silveri MC, Romani C, Caramazza A (1989) Variation in the pattern of omissions and substitutions of grammatical morphemes in the spontaneous speech of so-called agrammatic patients. Brain and Language 36: 447–92.

Miller G (1985) Dictionaries in the mind. Language and Cognitive Processes 3: 171–85.

Millis S, Button S (1989) The effect of polysemy on lexical decision time: now you see it, now you don't. Memory and Cognition 17, 141–7.

Mimouni Z, Jarema G (1997) Agrammatic aphasia in Arabic. Aphasiology 11: 125–44.

Moens M, Steedman M (1987) Temporal ontology in natural language. In 25th ACL Meeting, Stanford, CA, pp. 1–7.

Mohr J (1976) Broca's area and Broca's aphasia. In Whitaker H, Whitaker HA (eds) Studies in Neurolinguistics. New York: Academic Press.

Myerson R, Goodglass H (1972) Transformational grammars of three agrammatic patients. Language and Speech 15: 40–50.

Neely JH (1991) Semantic priming effects in visual word recognition: a selective review of current findings and theories. In Besner D, Humphreys GW (eds) Basic Processes in Reading: Visual Word Recognition. New Jersey: Lawrence Erlbaum Associates.

Nespoulous J-L, Dordain M, Perron C, Ska B, Bub D, Caplan D, Mehler J, Lecours AR (1988) Agrammatism in sentence production without comprehension deficits: reduced availability of syntactic structures and/or of grammatical morphemes? a case study. Brain and Language 33: 273–95.

Nespoulous J-L, Dordain M., Perron C, Jarema G, Chazal M (1990) Agrammatism in French: two case studies. In Menn L, Obler L (eds) Agrammatic Aphasia: A Cross-language Narrative Sourcebook. Philadelphia: John Benjamin's Publishing Company.

Nicol J (1988) Coreference processing during sentence comprehension. Unpublished doctoral dissertation, MIT, Cambridge, MA.

Nicol J, Swinney D (1989) The role of structure in coreference assignment during sentence comprehension. Journal of Psycholinguistic Research: Special Issue on Sentence Processing 18(1): 5–24.

Nicol J, Pickering M (1993) Processing syntactically ambiguous sentences: evidence from semantic priming. Journal of Psycholinguistic Research 22.

Nicol J, Fodor JD, Swinney D (1994) Using cross-modal lexical decision tasks to investigate sentence processing. Journal of Experimental Psychology: Learning, Memory, and Cognition 20(5): 1229–38.

Nicol J, Swinney D, Love T, Hald L (1997) Examination of sentence processing with continuous vs. interrupted presentation paradigms. Center for Human Information Processing, Technical report #97-3, UCSD, La Jolla, CA. 92093.

Osman-Sági J (1991) Az afázia klasszifikációja és diagnosztikéja [Diagnosis and classification of aphasia]. Ideggyógy·szati Szemle 44(8): 339–62.

Ouhalla J (1990) Sentential negation, relativised minimality and the aspectual status of auxiliaries. The Linguistic Review 7: 183–231.

Ouhalla J (1993) Functional categories, agrammatism and language acquisition. Linguistische Berichte 143: 3–36.

Partee B, Roth M (1983) Generalized conjunction and type ambiguity. In Meaning, Use and Interpretation of Language. Walter de Gruyter.

Perlmutter D, Rosen C (eds) (1984) Studies in Relational Grammar 2. Chicago: University of Chicago Press.

Pesetsky D (1987) Wh-in-situ: movement and unselective binding. In Ter Meulen A, Reuland E (eds) Representation of (in)definiteness. Cambridge, MA: MIT Press.

Piñango MM (1998) Syntactic and semantic operations and their neurological underpinnings. Dissertation, Brandeis University, Waltham, MA.

Pollock JY (1994) Checking theory and bare verbs. In Cinque G et al. (eds) Paths Towards Universal Grammar: Studies in Honor of Richard S. Kayne. Georgetown Studies in Romance Linguistics, pp. 293–308.

Prather P, Shapiro L, Zurif E, Swinney D (1991) Real-time examinations of lexical processing in aphasics. Journal of Psycholinguistic Research 20 (Special Issue on Sentence Processing): 271–81.

Pullum GK (1991) The Great Eskimo Hoax and Other Irreverent Essays on the Study of Language. Chicago: University of Chicago Press.

Pustejovsky J (1991) The generative lexicon. Computational Linguistics 17: 409–41.

Pustejovsky J (1995) The Generative Lexicon. Cambridge, MA: MIT Press.

Radford A (1988) Transformational Syntax. Cambridge: Cambridge University Press.

Rayner K, Carlson M, Frazier L (1983) The interaction of syntax and semantics during sentence processing: eye movements in the analysis of semantically biased sentences. Journal of Verbal Learning and Verbal Behavior 22: 358–74.

Rice M, Wexler K, Cleave P (1995) Specific language impairment as a period of extended optional infinitive. Journal of Speech and Hearing Research 38: 850–63.

Rizzi L (1990) Relativized Minimality. Cambridge, MA: MIT Press.

Rubin SS, Newhoff M, Peach RK, Shapiro LP (1996) Electrophysiological indices of lexical processing: the effects of verb complexity and age. Journal of Speech and Hearing Research 39: 1071–80.

Ruigendijk E, van Zonneveld R, Bastiaanse R (in press) Case assignment in agrammatism. Journal of Speech, Language and Hearing Disorders.

Saddy D (1995) Variables and events in the syntax of agrammatic speech. Brain and Language 50: 135–50.

Saffran EM, Schwartz MF, Marin OSM (1980) The word order problem in agrammatism: production. Brain and Language 10: 263–80.

Saffran EM, Berndt RS, Schwartz MF (1989) The quantitative analysis of agrammatic production: procedure and data. Brain and Language 37: 440–79.

Schwartz MF, Saffran EM, Marin OSM (1980) The word order problem in agrammatism: comprehension. Brain and Language 10, 249–62.

Schwartz MF, Linebarger M, Saffran EM, Pate D (1987) Syntactic transparency and sentence interpretation in aphasia. Language and Cognitive Processes 2: 85–113.

Sells P (1985) Lectures on Contemporary Syntactic Theories. Stanford, CA: CSLI.

Shapiro, LP (1997) Tutorial: an introduction to syntax. Journal of Speech, Language, and Hearing Research 40: 254–72.

Shapiro LP, Hestvik A (1995) On-line comprehension of VP-ellipsis: syntactic reconstruction and semantic influence. Journal of Psycholinguistic Research 24: 517–32.

Shapiro L, Levine B (1990) Verb processing during sentence comprehension in aphasia. Brain and Language 38: 21–47.

Shapiro LR, Zurif E, Grimshaw J (1987) Sentence processing and the mental representation of verbs. Cognition 27: 219–46.

Shapiro LR, Zurif E, Grimshaw J (1989) Verb representation and sentence processing: contextual impenetrability. Journal of Psycholinguistic Research 18: 223–43.

Shapiro LP, Brookins B, Gordon B, Nagel HN (1991) Verb effects during sentence processing. Journal of Experimental Psychology: Learning, Memory, & Cognition 17:

983–96.

Shapiro LR, Gordon B, Hack N, Killackey J (1993) Verb-argument structure processing in complex sentences in Broca's and Wernicke's aphasia. Brain and Language 45: 423–47.

Shapiro LP, Hestvik A, Suzuki E, Garcia R (1998) Verb properties and gap-filling in complex VP ellipsis constructions. Paper presented to the CUNY Human Sentence Processing Conference, New Jersey.

Shapiro LP, Swinney DA, Borsky S (1998) On-line examination of language performance in normal and neurologically-impaired adults. American Journal of Speech-Language Pathology 7: 49–60.

Shapiro LP, Oster E, Garcia AR, Massey A, Thompson (1999) Processing wh-questions: a time course analysis. Presentation of CUNY Human Sentence Processing Conference, New York.

Shlonsky U (1997) Clause Structure and Word Order in Hebrew and Arabic. New York: Oxford University Press.

Sportiche D (1988) A theory of floating quantifiers and its corollaries for constituent structure. Linguistic Inquiry 19: 425–49.

Stark J (1992) Everyday Life Activities: Photo Series. Vienna: Druckerei Bosmüller.

Stark JA, Dressler WU (1990) Agrammatism in German: two case studies. In Menn L, Obler L (eds) Agrammatic Aphasia: A Cross-language Narrative Sourcebook. Philadelphia: John Benjamin's Publishing Company.

Stowe LA (1986) Parsing WH-constructions: evidence for on-line gap location. Language & Cognitive Processes 1(3): 227–45.

Stromswold K, Caplan D, Alpert N, Rauch S (1996)Localization of syntactic comprehension by PET. Brain and Language 52: 452–73.

Swinney D (1979) Lexical access during sentence comprehension: (re) consideration of context effects. Journal of Verbal Learning and Verbal Behavior 18: 645–59.

Swinney D, Osterhout L (1990) Inference generation during auditory language comprehension. The Psychology of Learning 25: 17–33.

Swinney D, Osterhout L (1991) Inference generation during language comprehension. In Graesser A, Bower GH (eds) The Psychology of Learning and Motivation: Inference and Text Comprehension. New York: Academic Press.

Swinney D, Zurif EB (1995) Syntactic processing in aphasia. Brain and Language 50: 225–39.

Swinney D, Love T (1998) Language input rate as a parameter on structural processing. Proceedings of 11th Annual CUNY Conference on Human Sentence Processing, New Brunswick, NJ (March 1998).

Swinney D, Onifer W, Prather P, Hirshkowitz M (1979) Semantic facilitation across sensory modalities in the processing of individual words and sentences. Memory & Cognition 7(3): 159–65.

Swinney D, Ford M, Frauenfelder U, Bresnan J (1987) On the temporal course of gap-filling and antecedent assignment during sentence comprehension. In Grosz B, Kaplan R, Macken M, Sag I (eds) Language Structure and Processing, Stanford, CA: CSLI.

Swinney D, Zurif EB, Prather P, Love T (1996) Neurological distribution of processing operations underlying language comprehension. Journal of Cognitive Neuroscience 8(2):174–84.

Swinney D, Nicol J, Love T, Hald L (1998) Methodological issues in the on-line study of language processing. In Schwartz R (ed) Childhood Language Disorders. New Jersey: Lawrence Erlbaum Associates.

Tabossi P (1988) Accessing lexical ambiguities in different types of sentential contexts. Journal of Memory and Language 27: 324–41.

Tanenhaus MK, Leiman JM, Seidenberg MS (1979) Evidence for multiple stages in the processing of ambiguous words in syntactic contexts. Journal of Verbal Learning & Verbal Behavior 18(4): 427–40.

Tanenhaus MK, Carlson G, Seidenberg MS (1985) Do listeners compute linguistic representations? In Dowdy DR, Kartunnen L, Zwicky AM (eds) Natural Language Parsing: Psychological, Computational, and Theoretical Perspectives. New York: Cambridge University Press.

Tanenhaus MK, Stowe LA, Carlson G (1985) The interaction of lexical expectation and pragmatics in parsing filler-gap constructions. In Proceedings of the Seventh Annual Cognitive Science Meetings, pp. 361–5.

Tanenhaus MK, Carlson G, Trueswell JC (1989) The role of thematic structures in interpretation and parsing. Language and Cognitive Processes 4(SI): 211–34.

Thompson CK, Lange KL, Schneider SL, Shapiro LP (1997) Agrammatic and non-brain-damaged subjects' verb and verb argument structure production. Aphasiology 11: 473–90.

Thompson CK, Shapiro LP (1994) A linguistic-specific approach to treatment of sentence production deficits in aphasia. Clinical Aphasiology 22: 307–23.

Thompson CK, Shapiro LP (1995) Training sentence production in agrammatism: implications for normal and disordered language. Brain and Language 50: 201–24.

Thompson CK, Shapiro LP, Roberts MM (1993) Treatment of sentence production deficit in aphasia: a linguistic-specific approach to wh-interrogative training and generalization. Aphasiology 7: 111–33.

Thompson CK, Shapiro LP, Schneider S, Tait M (1994) Linguistically informed analysis of agrammatic aphasic language production. Paper presented at the TENET V Conference, Montreal, Canada.

Thompson CK, Shapiro LP, Li L, Schendel L (1995) Analysis of verbs and verb-argument structure: a method for quantification of aphasic language production. Clinical Aphasiology 23: 121–40.

Thompson CK, Shapiro LP, Tait ME, Jacobs MJ, Schneider SL (1996) Training wh-question production in agrammatic aphasia: analysis of argument and adjunct movement. Brain and Language 52: 175–228.

Thompson CK, Shapiro LP, Ballard KJ, Jacobs BJ, Schneider SS, Tait ME (1997) Training and generalized production of wh- and NP-movement structures in agrammatic aphasia. Journal of Speech, Language, and Hearing Research 40: 228–44.

Tissot R, Mounin G, Lhermitte F, Dordain G (1973) L'Agrammatisme. Brussels: Charles Dessart.

Trueswell JG, Tanenhaus MK, Garnsey SM (1994) Semantic influences on parsing: use of thematic role information in syntactic disambiguation. Journal of Memory and Language 33: 285–318.

Van Riemsdijk H, Williams E (1986) Introduction to the Theory of Grammar. Cambridge, MA: MIT Press.

Vermeulen J, Bastiaanse R, Wageningen B van (1989) Spontaneous speech in aphasia: a correlational study. Brain and Language 36: 252–74.

Vignolo L (1988) The anatomical and pathological basis of aphasia. In Rose FC, Whurr R, Wyke M (eds), Aphasia. London: Whurr.

Walenski M (1997) Compounding cues. Center for Human Information Processing. Technical report #97-5, UCSD, La Jolla, CA 92093.

Weinrich M, Shelton JR, Cox DM, McCall D (1997) Remediating production of tense morphology improves verb retrieval in chronic aphasia. Brain and Language 58: 23–45.

Wexler K (1994) Optional infinitives, head movement and the economy of derivations.

In Lightfoot D, Hornstein N (eds) Verb Movement. Cambridge: Cambridge University Press.

Whitworth A (1995a) Characterising thematic role assignment in aphasic sentence production: procedures for elicited and spontaneous output. European Journal of Disorders of Communication 30: 384–99.

Whitworth A (1995b) Thematic Roles in Production (TRIP): An Assessment of Word Retrieval at the Sentence Level. London: Whurr.

Williams SE, Canter GJ (1987) Action-naming performance in four syndromes of aphasia. Brain and Language 32: 124–36.

Woolford E (1991) VP-internal subjects in VSO and nonconfigurational languages. Linguistic Inquiry 2: 503–40.

Zaenen A, Maling J (1984) Unaccusative, passive and quirky case. In West Coast Conference on Formal Linguistics 3. U.C. Santa Cruz: Stanford Linguistics Association, pp. 317–29.

Zingeser LB, Berndt RS (1990) Retrievals of nouns and verbs in agrammatism and anomia. Brain and Language 39: 14–32.

Zurif E, Swinney D (1994) Neuropsychology of sentence comprehension. In Gernsbacher MA (ed) Handbook of Psycholinguistics. Orlando, FL: Academic Press.

Zurif EB, Swinney D, Prather P, Solomon J, Bushell C (1993) An on-line analysis of syntactic processing in Broca's and Wernicke's aphasia. Brain and Language 45: 448–64.

Zurif EB, Swinney D, Prather P, Wingfield A, Brownell H (1995) The allocation of memory resources during sentence comprehension: evidence from the elderly. Journal of Psycholinguistic Research 24: 165–82.

Zwart CJW (1993) Dutch syntax: a minimalist approach. Groningen Dissertations in Linguistics.

Index